Primary Healthcare Premises

An Expert Guide

SEAMUS KEHOE
LYNNE ABBESS
VALERIE MARTIN
NEIL NIBLETT
PETER STYLIANOU

FOREWORD BY
TONY STANTON

RADCLIFFE MEDICAL PRESS

© 1999 Seamus Kehoe

Radcliffe Medical Press Ltd
18 Marcham Road, Abingdon, Oxon OX14 1AA

British Library Cataloguing in Publication Data

A catalogue record for this book is available from the British Library.

ISBN 1 85775 122 1

Typeset by Acorn Bookwork, Salisbury, Wiltshire
Printed and bound by Biddles Ltd, Guildford and King's Lynn

Contents

Foreword

Good premises are essential to the delivery of high quality primary healthcare. The Government has brought forward detailed plans aimed at improving the quality of care provided to patients receiving NHS services. The initial delegation of some key functions of health authorities to primary care groups who have to deliver primary care investment plans is likely to stimulate a lot of hard thinking about primary care premises. This process is given an added emphasis by the general power that primary care trusts will have to acquire land and obtain their own premises.

Doctors have made major investments in surgery premises, particularly over the last 25 years. Many of those premises will need redevelopment or replacement and the health centre stock generally needs a great deal of improvement. Many other doctors are working in even older premises for which there have not been the resources available to bring them up-to-date.

Anyone who is planning or considering primary healthcare premises for the future will find this book an invaluable guide. All of the contributors are truly experts in their fields. Peter Stylianou, who sets the tone by giving the health authority's viewpoint, has a very considerable experience in helping doctors develop premises in a challenging inner city area. Neil Niblett is a very experienced architect who has successfully carried through a large number of surgery developments. Lynne Abbess from the solicitors

Hempsons, has an unparalleled experience of the legal aspects of surgery ownership and the often complex relationship with partnership agreements. Seamus Kehoe is an independent financial adviser who has helped many practices obtain the finance they need to carry through surgery projects to a successful conclusion. The accountant's viewpoint provided by Valerie Martin shows how the financial viability of any scheme can be analysed and deals with the complexities of taxation, VAT and other potential hazards.

For most doctors, developing new premises is a once in a professional lifetime challenge. There is no substitute for taking expert advice, and this book makes a splendid starting point.

Tony Stanton
Chair of the Practice Premises Sub Committee
of the GPC
Director GPFC Ltd
Secretary, London Local Medical Committees
March 1999

Preface

Anyone who has travelled down the path of building or refurbishing their surgery premises will probably agree that not only is it the single greatest financial commitment in a GP's life, but it can also be one of the most daunting. The timescale from initial conception to practical completion can be many years.

Primary Healthcare Premises: An Expert Guide was specifically written with the intention of providing guidance for GPs who are embarking on a surgery development. It will enable them to complete their project with minimal disruption to their daily medical routine. The book contains viewpoints of five specialists based on practical experience gained from many years working in their individual fields.

Whilst it is designed as an in-depth point of reference, it also simplifies the development process by pointing out the numerous pitfalls that need to be avoided. This ensures that a project reaches a satisfactory conclusion. It should be read as an adjunct to the Red Book as that is the oracle for interpretation purposes in the event of a dispute with a health authority.

The book's probable readership includes GPs, PCGs trainees, practice managers and advisors to the GP profession. However, if it helps the reader, who ever that may be, to achieve a better understanding of this specialist subject then the co-author's efforts will have been worthwhile.

Our thanks are extended to Dr Tony Stanton for his Foreword and all at Radcliffe Medical Press for their help and support throughout the duration of the book's development.

Seamus Kehoe
March 1999

About the authors

Lynne Abbess BA (Hons)
Partner and Head of Professional Services Department
Hempsons Solicitors
Covent Garden, London
Tel: 0171 836 0011

Seamus Kehoe ACII
Cost and Notional Rent Specialist
The Quadrant Group
Stanmore, Middlesex
Tel: 0171 625 9455

Valerie Martin BA FCA
Partner and National Director of Medical Services
Pannell Kerr Forster
Guildford, Surrey
Tel: 01483 564646

Neil Niblett AMIAS Tech RICS FFB MBIM
Principal in the firm of Neil Niblett and Associates
Architecture, Project and Building Cost Management
Abergavenny, Gwent
Tel: 01873 858831

Peter Stylianou BSc (Econ)
Capital Projects Manager
Lambeth, Southwark and Lewisham Health Authority
Tel: 0171 226 4110

1

The health authority's viewpoint

PETER STYLIANOU

Introduction

The purpose of this chapter is to summarise the main provisions for the acceptance of practice premises for reimbursement purposes, how payments are calculated, and the range of funding options that might be available to practices contemplating changes to their surgeries or relocating to new premises.

A key point for any practice to remember is to ensure that they receive clear advice and guidance from their health authority (HA) on premises matters, particularly when contemplating a development scheme. In addition to the range of factors to be considered (covered in detail in other chapters), it is the HA which is ultimately responsible for the acceptance of premises and authorisation of payments. Close liaison with appropriate HA officers is therefore essential to avoid misunderstandings and maximise the opportunities for successful development.

Doctors should not be put off from trying to improve their premises arrangements. This book attempts to cover the various aspects of premises development: legal aspects, tax implications, design issues, finance arrangements, the regulatory frameworks, etc. Taken together, it could all seem unduly daunting. However, good premises make good sense, not just for patients and services, but for the practitioners themselves and their staff. Despite the hurdles and challenges involved, with good preparation and advice there is much that can be achieved and enormous satisfaction to be gained from developing good primary care premises.

Paragraphs 51 and 56 of the Statement of Fees and Allowances (SFA) are the main sources of reference for the information that follows. However, it is not the intention of this chapter simply to rewrite the SFA in more user-friendly terms. Rather, the intention is to illustrate the main principles and processes involved and also to consider issues from a HA perspective.

HAs will have local strategies, including plans for primary care premises, which reflect local priorities and local objectives. It is important, therefore, that doctors are aware of the strategic context within which decisions are made and which affect the levels of reimbursement in relation to premises. Funding for premises development is generally cash-limited and therefore subject to the availability of funds, regardless of whether the budget is controlled by the HA or the primary care groups (PCGs). Doctors cannot and should not assume that funding will be readily available, even when an excellent premises schemes is presented. You will need to argue your case as to why the HA should allocate public funds to your project and how the proposed changes will benefit patient services. Even where a proposed development does not require a cash-limited input, HAs have to be satisfied that any additional payments are justified in the interests of the service. A better understanding of the 'system' should place you at an advantage in trying to secure funding for GP premises.

This is not an exhaustive examination of all the possible issues that can affect premises payments and premises development. However, this chapter will cover the principal areas that affect most GPs, most of the time. This should also be regarded as a guide only to the main provisions around practice premises. Always ensure that you obtain independent advice and the advice of your local HA in order properly to reflect local conditions and circumstances.

Primary care arrangements underwent a significant change with the launch of PCGs from 1 April 1999. Along with organisational change, there may be regulatory changes which affect the type of premises payments that apply. That said, the Department of Health has indicated that the cost rent and improvement grant schemes continue to operate and therefore remain relevant. What follows reflects the rules and regulations currently in place.

Rent and rates scheme

Eligibility criteria and acceptance of premises

There is just a brief reference to practice premises under the Terms of Service for doctors. Paragraph 27, 'Arrangements at practice premises', is as follows:

> *A doctor shall:*
>
> (a) *provide proper and sufficient accommodation at his practice premises having regard to the circumstances of each practice, and*
>
> (b) *shall, on receipt of a written request from the HA allow inspection of those premises at a reasonable time by a member or officer of the HA or LMC or both, authorised by the HA for the purpose.*

You could be forgiven for concluding that the requirements for premises arrangements are not particularly onerous, but as in most areas of public finance, the devil is in the detail, and you have to refer to the SFA for the extent of that detail. As mentioned in the introduction, HA strategy may also influence what can be accepted and, for what has already been accepted, what might be further developed.

Who qualifies for rent and rates?

Doctors on the medical list of a HA with more than 100 patients (or deemed to be building up to 100 patients) can qualify for payments under the rents and rates (R&R) scheme. That said, the accommodation needs to be accepted by the HA before payments can commence. This will involve an inspection from a HA representative and sometimes a local medical committee (LMC) member. Most doctors reading this will already have practice premises for which they receive some level of payment and, by definition, their premises have already been accepted. But this is a point where it is useful to remember paragraph 51.12 (a particular favourite with HA premises managers) which explains that continued acceptance of premises is not indefinite. If there is something fundamentally wrong with your surgery, you will need to address it sooner or later, or you may find that your level of reimbursement is abated or withheld altogether (*see* pp 11–12).

What qualifies for acceptance?

Essentially, premises need to meet minimum standards and be of sufficient size for the volume of activity taking place (the 'proper and sufficient accommodation' of the Terms of Service). They also need to be in the right location. If a practice in the heart of a housing estate approached their HA with a request to move to new premises which would be 'state of the art' in design terms, but were over two miles away, it could (quite rightly) expect to hear dissenting voices.

Premises can be separate buildings or form part of a residence and can be rented or owned by the doctor. Please note that where premises are owned or rented by a close relative of the doctor (spouse, child, parent, grandparent, brother or sister) the HA will regard the GP as being an owner-occupier.

Whatever the status, the HA must be satisfied that the doctor is making reasonable use of the accommodation for the provision of agreed general medical services (GMS).

These notes apply to all surgeries, whether main or branch.

Minimum standards

What are the minimum standards?

The SFA definition for minimum standards is given in paragraph 51.10 and reproduced in full in Appendix A.

By themselves, these criteria do not appear overly demanding or exhaustive. However, it is a useful exercise for practices to critically assess their existing premises against these guidelines to see how well they perform. Some problems or shortcomings are not immediately recognised until a review is undertaken.

There is now much more detailed guidance available on the standards of practice accommodation in the form of a 'Commentary' (*see* SFA para. 51.52.2) which supplements the minimum standards shown above, and this is covered on p.21.

The formal assessment of standards rests with the HA, which must try to do so in a consistent and fair fashion. This is not necessarily straightforward as it is difficult, for example, to define what constitutes 'adequate lighting'. But despite the difficulties, it is the job of the local HA to reach a view on this following an inspection.

Inspections

Under the Terms of Service, doctors are obliged to grant access to their surgeries for visits from HA officers and members, provided reasonable notice is given. For many HAs, two weeks would be deemed as reasonable and, indeed, most practices are happy to co-operate. However, you cannot unreasonably refuse access to your surgery as this could lead to service committee proceedings on a potential breach of service. Your HA may have a scheme of regular inspections in place or premises matters may be raised during an informal visit, leading subsequently to a more formal 'inspection'.

The aim of inspections is to ensure that premises standards are satisfactory and, where appropriate, to encourage improvements. In most cases, HAs will wish to work collaboratively with a practice to help address any problems or to develop a plan which will overcome the problems in the longer term. For example, this may involve working up a scheme for relocation to new premises altogether.

Range of mainstream payments available

Once accepted, the following reimbursements are available towards practice premises:

- reimbursement of rent to practices leasing their premises
- reimbursement of notional rents to practices owning their premises
- reimbursement of business rates relating to surgery accommodation
- reimbursement of water rates
- reimbursement of trade refuse charges
- reimbursement of cost rent (*see* p.13).

How is rent reimbursement calculated?

Whether you own or rent your premises, the HA will use information supplied by the local district valuer (DV) to determine the amount paid.

Owner-occupiers

Where premises are owned, the DV will calculate a notional rent. This is the equivalent of the current market rental value that the DV considers you could expect to pay if the premises were actually rented. This will be in relation to the practice accommodation accepted by the HA at the date of valuation. The DV will exclude any part of the building which is not directly used for practice purposes, but will include parking spaces for use by patients and by practitioners exclusively for practice purposes. Any rental received by the practice from a third party for use of the accepted accommodation will be deducted from the reimbursement made.

Tenants

Where premises are rented, the reimbursement will be the lesser of the actual rent paid by the practice or the DV's opinion of the current market rental value. Again, the valuation will be based on the accommodation that has been accepted by the HA under the scheme. Where payments for rent include VAT, this can be added to the reimbursement where it is properly charged to the practice by the landlord.

Separate premises

For separate premises, the accommodation must be self-contained and used by the practice. Optional rooms provided for attached community trust staff (e.g. health visitors) or local authority social workers can also be included. Practices can, in addition and at the discretion of the HA, provide more accommodation for community trust staff, in which case a rent will be payable by the trust (e.g. an office base for district nurses serving the locality). The practice, HA and trust will normally have to agree on the funding arrangements in such circumstances.

Surgeries forming part of a residence

For premises forming part of a residence, payments will relate solely to that part of the building used exclusively or primarily for practice purposes. For rooms used partly for practice and non-practice purposes, an apportionment may be applied.

What is the role of the district valuer?

The valuation office is an executive agency of the Inland Revenue and has a number of local district valuation offices to cover different areas. (HAs may have more than one DV office within their borders.) The DV provides a range of premises-related advice to HAs and assesses all the current market rent of surgeries and the gross value for rating purposes. The DV is provided with details of the practice accommodation as given on form PREM 1, completed by the doctors. It is often necessary for the DV to carry out a practice visit before issuing a report and it is in doctors' interests to provide access as soon as possible.

HAs cannot reimburse more than the level as advised by the DV. In reaching his opinion the DV takes account of a number of factors: location, amount of accommodation, the terms of a lease where that applies or is deemed to apply. For full details, please refer to paragraph 51/Schedule 4 of the SFA.

Can doctors dispute the HA's level of reimbursement?

Representations can be made against levels of rent reimbursement. As a tenant, you may find that your landlord seeks to charge a rent which is higher than that which the DV considers appropriate. In such circumstances the HA will pay the lower figure and the practice will be responsible for the difference. It may be possible to negotiate with the landlord to bring the rent into line with the opinion of the DV. Alternatively, you can submit independent evidence to the HA to be passed on to the DV in support of a higher assessment. In some cases, it may be possible for the DV to negotiate directly with your landlord to reach an agreed figure, but you will need to liaise with your HA to establish whether this can be done.

Similarly, if you are an owner-occupier and consider the notional rent to be low, you can submit independent evidence via the HA to the DV for his or her reconsideration. The DV may be prepared to reopen negotiations with the practice or its advisors with a view to reaching an agreement on the appropriate level of reimbursement.

In either case, 'independent evidence' normally requires a case prepared by a surveyor or valuer appointed by the practice for that purpose, the cost of which has to be met by the doctors.

Business rates, water rates and trade refuse charges

All practice accommodation is liable for business and water rates. Where premises have been accepted for rent purposes, reimbursement of business and water rates also applies.

Business and water rates (whether metered or standard) are reimbursed in full, subject to any necessary apportionment for non-practice accommodation.

Practices usually claim reimbursement after they have paid their bills and submitted their receipts to the HA. However, many HAs now have systems in place where, with the agreement of the GPs, the rates are paid direct to the charging authorities concerned, thus reducing paperwork considerably. Details of any payments made in this way should still be available to GPs for entry into the practice accounts. Please check with your HA to see what system of reimbursement is in place.

Many surgeries are charged trade refuse fees by their local authority and where this is the case, appropriate receipts can be submitted for reimbursement by the HA. Alternatively, you can be reimbursed the cost of suitable and cheaper alternative arrangements provided by another contractor.

How might private income affect rent and rates reimbursement?

If a practice uses its premises for work generating private income (defined as all professional income received other than from public sources), the rent and rates reimbursement paid may be abated. However, provided gross receipts from private work account for less than 10% of the total gross receipts for the practice, there will be no abatement. If private income is between 10% and 20% of the gross receipts, then an abatement of 10% will be made to reimbursements; if between 20% and 30% of gross receipts, then a 20% abatement will be made; and so on.

Claims for payment

Where premises have been accepted, doctors are required to submit a form PREM 1. This form is issued in triplicate and one copy should be retained by the practice, whilst the other two are returned to the HA. The aim of the form is to obtain details from doctors concerning the type of premises they have, the range of accommodation and other details, such as lease arrangements. Always contact the HA prior to completion where there are any doubts concerning what is required. A copy of the PREM 1 is forwarded to the DV when a formal rent assessment is required.

A PREM 1 form must be completed where there are new premises, changes to existing premises, or it is time for a notional rent review.

In addition, an annual claim form in respect of all premises, PREM 2, must be submitted within seven days of 30 June. This form includes a declaration from the practice concerning its income from private earnings and is valid for the subsequent 12 months. Doctors should return this form promptly, as failure to do so may lead to delays in payment.

Payments of notional rent are normally paid automatically (quarterly or monthly, subject to prior arrangement with the HA). For rented accommodation, rates and other charges, reimbursement will be made upon production of the appropriate receipts (unless payments are made direct: *see* business rates section above).

Review arrangements

Regular reviews

The scheme provides for regular reassessment of reimbursements to keep pace with market prices. For owner-occupiers, the DV will be asked to reassess the notional rent every three years. Shortly before the review is due, the HA will ask the practice to complete a PREM 1 form. This should show the current usage of accommodation. If there are any changes from the previous PREM 1, you can expect the HA to query the difference if it is unaware of any changes. The form is then sent to the DV for his or her opinion of current market rental value. It should be noted that there is no guarantee that the new notional rent will be higher than the previous figure, as the assessment is based on market prices.

For rented accommodation, a review is triggered when the landlord seeks to alter the actual rent. The terms and review mechanisms for this will be contained within the lease and typically occur every three or five years. A PREM 1 should be completed, or if there have been no changes since the last review apart from the level of rent itself, a simpler form, PREM 1A, can be submitted. The DV will assess whether the rent the practice is being charged is reasonable in the light of current market trends.

It may be that your premises are altered between normal reviews. For example, you may wish to bring into practice use a room not normally used, or you may have built an extension to create additional accommodation.

In the normal course of events, practices will liaise closely with their HA prior to any such changes to establish whether the proposals can be accepted under the scheme. Where changes have been approved, a review will take place with a new valuation date determined by the day that the changes were completed. Thereafter, for owner-occupiers, the date for reviewing the current market rent will be every three years on the anniversary of the new assessment.

Reviews following concerns over minimum standards

The level of reimbursements can also be reviewed where there are concerns regarding the standard of the premises. It is within the HA's remit to review the payments following an inspection, and paragraph 51.12 of the SFA states, *inter alia*:

> ...*where the HA is of the view, following a visit, that any premises accepted under the Scheme are failing to meet these guidelines and it is reasonable to expect the practitioner to put the shortcomings right, the HA may, after consultation with the LMC, give notice to the practitioner concerned that payments of rent and rates under the Scheme will cease or be abated until it is satisfied that the shortcomings in the premises have been put right or will have been put right within a reasonable time. Any such notice will not have effect until 6 calendar months from the date on which it is issued.*

If the HA, after consultation with the LMC, comes to the conclusion that there are shortcomings with the premises, it can issue a notice to the practice to explain the problems and the implications if they are not rectified.

The HA should clearly set out in writing the list of things which are considered unacceptable and indicate what needs to be done to redress the problems within a reasonable time frame. If this is not made clear, you should ensure that it is explained properly to you.

For example, a HA may write to say that disabled access and facilities must be provided within six months, or it will abate future levels of reimbursement. It is also possible for HAs to institute service committee proceedings if the failings within the premises are such that they are considered a potential breach of the Terms of Service.

Whilst the HA has powers to restrict payments or remove them altogether, its powers to close down surgeries are restricted (although the Health and Safety Executive can close premises if they pose a health and safety risk to the public). Few authorities would wish to place pressure on a practice to close its premises unless and until there was somewhere better for patients to go. A collaborative approach is preferred whereby options for improvement are explored. After all, some funding may even be available to assist in rectifying the shortcomings.

Can doctors appeal against a notice of abatement?

Doctors have the right of appeal under paragraph 80.1 against any decision affecting applications or claims and this is no exception. If you wish to appeal, you should do so in writing to the Secretary of State within two calendar months, setting out your reasons for appeal.

The experience of this writer is that improvement notices are not issued lightly and it is not usually enough to try to argue that your premises have previously been accepted for many years. The role of HAs has changed since the time of Family Practitioner Committees, as too has surgery design to reflect the changing role of general practice. HAs have a duty to ensure that minimum standards are met in the interest of patients and will pay more attention to quality issues than perhaps they did in the past.

Doctors are ultimately responsible for their premises. Whether funding and support is made available or not, it is up to practitioners to ensure that their premises are meeting minimum standards and complying with their Terms of Service. The subsequent sections explore the principal methods of funding that may be available to assist practices in developing their surgeries.

Financial accounting

It is worth noting how HAs account for the payments they make and how this may affect the decision-making process. At the time of writing, rent and rates reimbursements are accounted for as GMS non cash-limited payments. HAs must ensure that all such payments are appropriate and in the interests of the service as a whole.

The same applies to cost rents and improvement grants, although there is an added dimension in that these reimbursements must be managed within a HA's annual cash-limited GMS budget.

HAs are mindful that all premises-related payments are financed by the taxpayer and reimbursements for GP surgeries must be justified at all times.

Cost rent scheme

Introduction

A detailed description of the cost rent scheme is contained in paragraphs 51.50 to 51.60 of the *Red Book,* covering some 40 pages, plus schedules. It does not necessarily make for easy reading and as a consequence, the cost rent scheme has acquired something of a mystique about it. It has also come in for criticism for having out-of-date schedules and constituting a high-risk approach. In some quarters, cost rent has not been encouraged at all.

But reports of the demise of the cost rent scheme are somewhat exaggerated. Indeed, the scheme has had something of a rebirth recently, with new arrangements issued by the Department of

Health which came into effect on 1 November 1997. The changes address many of the criticisms associated with the original scheme, which dates back to 1966, since when it has been considered 'past its sell-by date' by many commentators. The guidance in this section is based on the new cost rent schedules and amendments.

Cost rent is not as complicated as it may first appear. Neither does it need to be an unduly risky venture. In some instances it may be one of the few tools available to tackle more substantial and ambitious projects. This method of reimbursement can be a very suitable vehicle for creating purpose-built practice premises or their equivalent when properly researched and considered. But it does have its constraints, not least whether funding is available. The new cost rent provisions are welcomed in that they may alleviate some of the long-standing constraints. As an option for improving primary care buildings, doctors and HAs should not be deterred in considering and pursuing a cost rent scheme as a potential solution.

How does cost rent work?

In the previous section, we saw how market prices affected the level of rent payments and how the DV plays a pivotal role in determining the amount of reimbursement. Cost rent employs an entirely different method in arriving at the level of payment and is designed to encourage the improvement of the general standard of surgery premises.

It differs from current market rent in that payments are calculated as a percentage of the actual costs of developing a new or substantially modified surgery, subject to certain allowances, and can be applied to a variety of different models to reflect various circumstances and situations.

In effect, it is designed to reimburse the loan interest of providing new premises or substantial modification of an existing building. A simplified example is given in Box 1.1 to illustrate this principle.

This is a simplified example to illustrate the principles behind cost rent reimbursement and how this differs from current market rent. In practice, there are many variations from this example, but

Box 1.1:   Example of the cost rent scheme

Practice A currently works from cramped sub-standard accommodation which they rent from the local council. The HA reimburses the rent in full (the amount having been agreed by the district valuer), but there is a recognition that new premises are required for the long term.

The practice identifies a site nearby and investigates the feasibility of moving into new, purpose-built accommodation which they will own. The estimated cost of purchasing the site, constructing the surgery, the professional, statutory and legal fees, plus VAT, is £655 000. The practice would therefore need to raise this sum and pay off the loan over a period of time. The interest to be paid on the loan will be £65 000 pa.

As owners, Practice A would be entitled to notional rent payments. However, the DV considers that the proposed new surgery will generate a notional rent of £40 000 pa. There is little incentive therefore for the practice to proceed on this basis.

Under the cost rent scheme, payments are based on a percentage of the applicable 'cost rent limit'. This is a formula which takes account of the cost of purchasing land, construction, fees, etc. In this example, Practice A's cost rent limit is £652 970 and the prescribed percentage is 10%, resulting in payments of £65 297 pa. This therefore offers a far greater incentive and almost meets the cost of paying the interest.

the essential theme is that payments are related more to the capital costs of the project rather than the current market rental value of the end product.

The cost rent scheme can be used for:

- new premises to be owned by the practice or rented from a third party
- premises bought for substantial modification
- substantial modification of existing premises owned by the practice or rented from a third party
- practices wishing to develop purpose-built premises or their equivalent for subsequent purchase and leaseback by a third party.

Applying for a cost rent

The first step is to approach your HA on an informal basis to discuss your ideas in outline. The purpose of this is to ascertain the general level of support that is likely to be available for your proposal. Questions to be tackled early on include: does the HA agree that you need better premises? Do you need to move or can you develop the existing surgery? What is the general funding situation? What guidance, advice and support is available from the HA? Are there alternative mechanisms to consider which might be more suitable?

An informal view of the proposals and the likely timetable for funding can thus be obtained, but the practice should then make a formal application. This will take the form of a written request (or a format as required by the local HA). Doctors need to check with their HA as to what arrangements apply locally.

Your application, in whatever format, should detail the shortcomings of your existing surgery arrangements and your arguments for a new or improved surgery. It is helpful to provide HAs with a service development plan to show how the range and quality of services for patients might improve if you had better facilities and more space.

The HA considers the application in relation to its Health Improvement Programme, its general policy for surgery improvements and its cash allocation. It has to consider whether the additional expenditure incurred by making a cost rent payment is warranted in terms of an improved service to patients. Factors to be taken into account include the number of patients registered with the practice, their geographical spread, an assessment of local health needs, the relation of the proposed premises to surrounding practices, including any other ongoing developments, whether the practice is a training practice, and so on.

Whilst you will not necessarily need architects drawings or costings etc. at this stage, you should provide details of the proposed location. Your initial aim is to obtain approval in principle, and based on the information above and the supporting details submitted by the practice, the HA will decide whether to grant outline approval under the cost rent scheme. You should ensure that outline approval is obtained in writing prior to undertaking more detailed (and potentially costly) work.

Always check to see whether your HA can offer more direct

support and advice. It is in your interests to establish at the outset what help is available and on what conditions.

HA cash limits for surgery improvements

Since April 1990, HAs have been allocated cash limits from which they reimburse all existing cost rents and meet the cost of new schemes. (The cash limits also cover improvement grants, practice staff budgets, staff training and practice computers.) The HA has therefore to look very carefully at every application and in giving outline approval bear in mind its own policies and priorities. The authority will be able to give an informal indication of whether a project will fall within its premises investment programme and the year within which cash may become available.

Cost rent projects are likely to take a considerable time and once the details of outline approval are known the practice will need to timetable the project accordingly. Almost invariably things happen which change the actual finishing date for the building or affect costs or both. The authority must be kept fully informed so that it can consider any changes in the light of its resources. Do not assume that the HA can automatically absorb increased costs due to variations from a previously agreed plan.

From 1 April 1999 with the introduction of PCGs, control over cash-limited budgets is likely to change although the pace of change from one PCG to another may vary. As PCG structures and management arrangements take shape and mature, it is likely that more and more responsibility for targeting cash-limited resources against premises schemes will shift to PCGs. The key point for practices to bear in mind, regardless of where budgetary control ultimately lies, is that resources are limited and applications for funding need to demonstrate that they fit in with local priorities and provide good value for money.

Type of cost rent

There are several types of project which may qualify for cost rent reimbursement, each involving a different method of calculation. These are summarised as follows:

- **New premises owned by the practice:** these are schemes where the practice purchases a site and builds new, separate premises.
- **New premises rented by the practice:** these are new purpose-built premises developed by a third party and leased to the practice.
- **Premises bought for substantial modification:** these are premises not previously owned by the practice which are bought and substantially modified to provide the equivalent of purpose-built accommodation.
- **Substantial modification of existing premises owned by the practice:** these are schemes where the practice substantially modifies its existing premises to provide the equivalent of purpose-built accommodation.
- **Substantial modification of existing premises not owned by the practice:** these are schemes which involve the substantial modification of existing premises which are owned by a third party. The alterations are undertaken by the landlord and a new lease and rental are agreed.
- **Purchase and lease:** these are projects in which banks, building societies or other reputable financial institutions acquire from a practice newly completed, purpose-built premises or their equivalent and lease them back to the practice.

Although no precise definition of 'substantial modification' is given in the SFA, such alterations must involve structural work, by extension to or internal modification of a building.

Your HA can guide you through this definition and explain whether your proposals constitute a substantial alteration/modification.

The process: general guidance

Having obtained outline approval, you need to undertake a more detailed investigation of the proposed scheme and assess the implications. This will require consideration of a number of factors.

Professional advice

Sound professional advice throughout is absolutely crucial to the success of your scheme and the selection of a good architect is essential. It is often helpful to talk to colleagues who have undertaken surgery developments about architects they have engaged and might recommend. Some HAs keep lists of approved architects, or can put you in touch with firms with relevant experience. If you are unsure which architect to choose, you should consider arranging interviews to help you decide. If the project proceeds, you can expect to have a long and close relationship with the architect for the duration and it is vital that you have a good working relationship based on mutual trust.

Once appointed, the architect will usually advise you further regarding the other professionals you are likely to need, such as a quantity surveyor and planning supervisor. You may also need a structural engineer, mechanical engineer and so on depending on the nature of the project. As the client, you will have the final say on who is appointed and on what terms. There are, of course, other areas where advice will be relevant, such as financial advice, legal advice, tax advice, etc., and these are covered in more detail elsewhere in this book.

Design

Good design is about delivering the type of building required to reflect your practice's needs, as well as complying with regulations and minimum standards. Wherever possible, flexibility should be built in to allow your building to adapt and grow should changes occur in the future. Remember, attractive design features often come at a price and you need to balance aesthetic objectives against financial realities. Chapter 2 covers the area of design in detail.

Meeting the cost rent standards

To succeed, you will need to produce plans which are acceptable to your local HA. Reference should be made to *General Medical*

Premises: a commentary, a guide published at the same time as the new cost rent schedule. This provides advice to HAs, GPs, their architects and other professionals on the development of high-quality premises, regardless of the funding arrangements. It includes guidance on design principles, space planning, additional facility areas, fabric and environment. A copy of this must be made available to your architects at the outset to ensure that their work is consistent with requirements. The HA will need to be convinced that your cost rent proposals meet these guidelines for the project to proceed.

Cost rent schedules

The new cost rent schedules, effective from 1 November 1997, set out the parameters for cost rent schemes, defining the gross internal areas and cost allowances for each size of development. These are set out in Schedule 1a (premises for one to five GPs) and Schedule 1b (premises for six to 10 GPs).

Two tables are used. Table 1.1 provides details of the maximum floor areas which apply. These areas are deemed sufficient to provide the range of facilities common to all practices for the delivery of modern general medical services. Table 1.2 provides for further areas to be incorporated in a cost rent project to meet the agreed needs of individual practices. The tables from Schedule 1a are reproduced here for illustration. (These figures will be reviewed regularly, so check with the HA to ensure that your information is up to date.)

For example a surgery to accommodate four GPs (referred to as a '4 dr unit') has an area allowance of $476\,m^2$, with a maximum basic building allowance of £341 000. To this allowance, the HA may approve additions to reflect agreed additional facilities (using Table 1.2), such as parking and external works, special site conditions, VAT and so on.

You should discuss the need for additional accommodation and demonstrate that services could not be provided within the standard area allowance. A practice service development plan is a useful tool to demonstrate the range of proposed services, facil-

Table 1.1: Gross internal areas and national building cost allowances

Number of GPs	1	2	3	4	5
Type of premises	A	A	A	B	B
Gross internal area (GIA) allowance, m^2	148	239	348	476	540
Building allowance, £	124 500	197 000	273 500	341 000	381 000
Car park, £	8600	16 000	22 600	28 300	33 300

ities, staff and anticipated developments in support of such discussions.

Cost rent premises should be built as close as possible to the limits. If new premises are built significantly smaller (i.e. more than 2.5% smaller) the maximum cost rent payable will be reduced proportionately for the total m^2 reduction that is made. If the premises are larger than the approved schedule size limits, the HA will not be able to increase the allowance on that account.

Table 1.2: Additional facilities – gross internal areas and national building allowances at £/m^2

Number of GPs	1	2	3	4	5
Building cost allowance, £/m^2	793	766	717	702	692
Practice manager, m^2	14	N/A	N/A	N/A	N/A
Part time GP, m^2	18	18	18	18	18
GP trainer, additional space, m^2	4	4	4	4	4
Medical trainees, m^2	18	18	18	18	18
Dispensary, m^2	14	14	23	23	23
Services management, m^2	16	16	24	24	32
Services development, m^2	16	16	34	44	54
Professional fees, %	12.5	12.4	12.3	12.2	12.1

District valuer

New premises

If the project involves the purchase of a site, the HA can obtain an assessment from the DV of the open market value of that site (including VAT where that properly applies). In order to do this the DV will require a site plan showing the boundaries of the site (preferably an Ordnance Survey plan). The DV's site value can then be used by the HA in its interim cost rent calculation and can advise practices accordingly as to the viability of the scheme. You will want to ensure that the price you pay for the site is as close as possible to the DV's opinion, as the cost rent always adopts the lesser of either the actual price paid or the DV's opinion of value. Check with the HA to establish whether the DV can negotiate the price directly with the vendor.

Substantial modification

If the project involves purchasing premises for substantial modification, the DV will be asked to assess the current market value of (i) the site alone and (ii) the premises including the site.

If existing premises of the practice are to be modified, the DV will be asked for an assessment of the current market value of the site of the premises when originally acquired by the practice, and will also be asked to provide a reassessment of the current market rent of the existing premises on the date that the practice accepts the tender for the work.

These assessments are used to calculate interim cost rents, according to the type of project involved.

Acquisition of land

Practices should not acquire land on a speculative basis, in the hope that cost rent approval will follow, or that the level of cost rent, where offered, will be sufficient to cover costs. Approval in principle does not constitute a formal offer and that will follow only once more details are obtained. You should therefore defer purchasing a site until a formal written offer is obtained, planning permission is in place and the financial implications fully assessed. Ideally, the purchase should take place shortly before construction is due to start.

Planning permission

New buildings and most substantial modifications will require planning permission. Where this is the case, it is helpful if you can engage the support of your HA when submitting a planning application. Copies of relevant planning permission will need to be .sent to your HA.

Terminating an existing lease

If your proposals involve surrendering an existing lease in order to relocate, the HA may be able to assist with the cost. From 1 April 1998 the HA may provide assistance as follows. Either:

- reimbursement of all or part of the cost agreed with the landlord to surrender the lease or to assign the interest in the property to another party; and reasonable legal costs, or
- continued reimbursement of all or part of the rent and rates of the leased premises where a surrender or assignment has not been possible. This is only available where the unexpired period on the current lease is five years or less.

Please note these new rules apply only where the existing premises are inadequate and the practice agrees to move to suitable alternative premises leading to service improvement agreed with the HA.

Reimbursement of surrender or assignment costs must be paid from cash-limited funds, so the HA will have regard to the availability of resources. The DV will also be asked for his/her opinion of the cost-effectiveness of surrender, assignment or continued lease payments.

Details are contained in paragraph 55 of the SFA.

Interim cost rent

After approval in principle, production of plans and DV assessments, the HA should be in a position to produce an interim cost rent and confirm whether it continues to support the scheme. It will do this in writing, setting out the method of calculation and the likely, or estimated, level of cost rent, based on the information available at that time. Of necessity it will employ allowances and prescribed percentages that apply at the time of writing.

This is unlikely to produce the final cost rent that will apply on completion of the project, but it will give a good indication of the likely payments and clearly indicate the method of calculation, showing where variables might occur. This should then enable the practice, taking the advice of its financial advisors as necessary, to judge whether the scheme is financially viable or can be made so by amendment.

Method of calculation

We have seen that there are different types of project available and each one is calculated in a different way, the precise basis of which is set out in the SFA. Details of the various calculations are given in paragraphs 51.53.1 to 51.58.18.

All the methods involve a calculation of a maximum cost rent limit, applying a prescribed percentage to the total.

Prescribed percentage

The prescribed percentage is an interest rate determined by the Department of Health and supplied to HAs. Two rates are set: a fixed interest rate and a variable rate. The former is set every quarter and the latter annually on 1 April. The rate used by the HA will depend on the type of scheme and the basis of the practice's loan.

Owner-occupiers

For schemes which will be owned by the practice, the prescribed percentage used will be fixed if the loan is wholly or mainly financed under a fixed rate (or if financed by the practice's own money). The HA will apply the percentage in force on the date that the tender for the work is accepted. If a variable rate loan is chosen, then the variable prescribed percentage is applied.

If the prescribed percentage used is the variable rate, the final cost rent paid by the HA will vary in line with any changes in the annual rate, whereas a practice receiving reimbursement based on a fixed rate will have its cost rent fixed for the duration of the loan (unless it has an option to switch its loan to variable rate, in which case reimbursement changes to variable also).

Tenants

If a practice is leasing premises from a third party, the prescribed percentage used will be the fixed rate prevailing at the time that the lease for the premises is signed.

General

Practices qualifying for reimbursement based on a fixed interest rate must apply in writing to the authority before the date the tenders are accepted, confirming the basis of financing the scheme. If the financial arrangements have not been finalised by then, the outline intentions must be notified to the HA before that date and confirmed as soon as possible, certainly within six months. In default of a proper notification, the variable prescribed percentage will be applied to the cost rent reimbursement.

Location factor

A location factor is also applied to the basic allowances to reflect differential building costs across the country. These are shown in the SFA at paragraph 51/Schedule 3.

Exceptional site costs

HAs have discretion to allow additional costs to reflect any special circumstances concerning the site that is being developed, if that site is the only option. For example, you may be obliged to take a site that requires additional foundation works because it is on a gradient. Or the local authority may insist that the finishes for the building are of a specified type costing more than that which you would normally incur in order to comply with local planning requirements.

Where exceptional site costs are anticipated, you should notify the HA at an early stage. The allowances that may be agreed will typically be based on the extra, additional cost that is deemed to be incurred as a result of the circumstances of the site, over and above those costs that would normally be expected.

Interest

Prior to the completion of works, the practice will normally need to draw down on its loan facility to pay for things such as purchase of the land and stage payments to the contractor and various professionals.

Under the scheme, the interest that accrues on these payments can be included in the calculation, subject to written confirmation from the bank of the amount that has accrued ('rolled-up interest') up to the date of completion.

Calculation of a cost rent

Taking the above notes into consideration, we can illustrate how a calculation is made. The example in Box 1.2 builds on that shown on p.15.

At interim cost rent stage, there will be elements that are estimates and some items that are unknown. But the practice can gauge the likely level of reimbursement against the likely costs as estimated by the architect and quantity surveyor. Practice A anticipates a total cost (excluding interest) of approximately £655 000 and will make a decision by comparing allowances with costs.

Please note that the cost rent scheme will not cover the cost of loose furniture or equipment and the financing of these needs to be

Box 1.2:   Interim cost rent for Practice A

Practice A intends to purchase a site and construct a 4 dr unit. It is a teaching practice based in an area with a location factor of 1.14. The gross internal area for the proposed plans is 494 m^2. The area allowance for a 4 dr unit is 476 m^2, but the HA has agreed to additional facilities of 18 m^2 for medical trainees.

The site and plans have been approved in principle by the HA and the cost of purchasing the site is £60 000. The DV has considered the value of the site and places a current market value which agrees with the actual price.

Car parking facilities will be included on site, for which the HA has agreed to accept the costs up to the limits allowed.

(Rates applicable @ 1.11.97)

(i)	4 dr unit (476 m^2)	341 000
	Car parking allowance	28 300
		369 300
(ii)	Additional facilities (18 m^2 × 702)	12 636
		381 936
(iii)	Location factor (× 1.14) =	435 407
(iv)	Professional fee allowance (12.2%)	53 120
		488 527
(v)	Exceptional site costs	12 000
		500 527
(vi)	VAT (17.5%)	87 592
		588 119

continued

(vii)	Statutory fees	2500
	Off-site costs/other allowable fees	2351
		592970
(viii)	Interest	Not known
(ix)	Site value	60000
	Total	652970
	Prescribed percentage (fixed @ 10%)	= £65297 pa

considered. Also, cost rent calculations represent a maximum allowance or limit. If the total actual costs are less than the cost rent limit, reimbursement is made on the basis of the lower, actual costs.

Proceeding with the scheme

If you decide to proceed, you are ready to go to tender stage. A minimum of three tenders is required, although the architect may recommend more. In exceptional circumstances, the HA may be prepared to accept fewer than three tenders, but you are always advised to obtain at least three to ensure that you have a range of bids to get the best price possible.

The HA may also ask for a copy of the Bill of Quantities or Specification of Works. These constitute a detailed breakdown of the works and enable the HA to examine which elements, if any, may be excluded for cost rent purposes. This may be relevant in the case of modifying an existing building for which there might be some element of repair or maintenance. Your HA will provide guidance in individual cases.

If the lowest tender proves higher than the level anticipated, you may have to consider amending your scheme in some way. You will certainly need to explore the implications with the HA, who can offer advice as to what might be possible. Assuming the tenders are acceptable, you are ready to proceed. You must advise the HA of the date on which the tender has been accepted and the projected completion date.

During the course of the works, you must notify the HA of any significant variations which affect either the cost of the scheme or the projected completion date. Keep a clear record of payments made and ensure that receipts are kept safely for subsequent submission to the HA after the project is completed.

Payment

Cost rent reimbursement does not commence until after the project has been completed and comes into practice use. When the work is finished, the practice must send to the HA receipted accounts for all work carried out. This is not necessarily as onerous as it sounds. Architects' interim certificates will have been issued during the course of the contract and receipts issued. (The HA may have asked for certificates to be copied to them during the construction phase.) The architect can also prepare a final account for the scheme along with the certificate of practical completion.

Copies of receipts for professional fees, legal accounts, statutory fees, etc. should be sent to the authority. A statement should also be obtained from the bank to confirm the amount of interest that has been incurred up to the date of completion.

Not all of the bills will have been fully paid by the completion date. For example, it is standard to retain a small percentage of the payments due to the main contractor for a period of time. This 'retention fee' will not be paid to the builder for at least six months after the date of practical completion.

However, the HA will not expect the practice to wait until all bills have been paid before commencing payments. Rather, it will commence interim payments based on the information available at the time. Eventually, with all bills paid and details submitted to the HA, a final cost rent will be issued and any necessary adjustments made, backdated to the commencement of payment.

When does cost rent payment commence?

This will normally be the date on the architect's completion certificate or the date the practice moved into the new premises, whichever is the later. The HA will wish to inspect the premises prior to payment.

Payments to the practice may be monthly or quarterly (please liaise with the HA to confirm local arrangements). They may be paid into your practice account or some other account as specified by the practice and agreed by the HA.

Notional rent reviews

Cost rent is designed to offer a better return than current market rent, and this tends to be the case for most developments at the outset.

For owner-occupiers, you may request a review of the current market rent every three years from the date that cost rent commenced. There may come a point, on a review, when the notional rent exceeds the level of cost rent that you receive. In this case, you have the option of switching the method of reimbursement from cost rent to notional rent. Once switched, you cannot return to cost rent payment.

Final cost rent calculation

Because of the different types of project that are possible and the consequent variations in the cost rent calculation that can apply, it is not possible to describe every scenario in detail. GPs should refer to the relevant section of the SFA which describes the nature of their scheme. Details for the procedures involved in each case can be found at paragraphs 51.54.1 to 51.58.21.

The final cost rent will be calculated in accordance with the provisions of the appropriate paragraph and doctors will be issued with written confirmation once all the relevant details have been received from the practice. The final cost rent applies from the agreed date for the commencement of reimbursement, so there may be arrears due (or recovery of overpayment) to cover any interim period.

Representations

If you are not satisfied with the final cost rent calculation and are unable to resolve matters with the HA, you can make representations to the Secretary of State within two months of the HA's decision.

The improvement grant scheme

Introduction

The improvement grant scheme is a relatively straightforward reimbursement system designed to provide a financial contribution towards the cost of carrying out approved improvements to surgery premises.

Essentially, practices can claim a contribution from the HA towards a range of surgery improvements, where these have received the prior approval of the authority. The level of grant offered can vary from 33% to 66% and is at the discretion of the HA. The grant can be applied to the cost of the approved work, including professional fees, local authority fees and VAT.

As with other SFA payments, there are eligibility criteria which must be met and an application process whereby the HA considers what funding might be appropriate.

Paragraph 56 of the SFA lays out the criteria which apply. This should be seen in the context of the HA's local policies and priorities, since the level and type of support available will vary from one area to another and be influenced by the availability of funds at the disposal of the HA.

Within London, practices falling within the 'London Initiative Zone' (LIZ) had access to additional support (the *enhanced improvement grant scheme*', which offered up to 90% grants), but these arrangements expired on 31 March 1999. Mainstream GMS improvement grants will continue to have a limit of 66% nationally from 1 April 1999.

Eligibility criteria

The principal criteria are:

- list size
- minimum cost of project
- eligible types of work
- security of tenure
- NHS use.

List size

To be eligible to receive a grant, a doctor should be providing unrestricted general medical services and have a list of 500 or more patients (or an average of 500 for partnerships). There is some flexibility on the list threshold if the HA considers that the practice will build up its list size to the relevant numbers over the next year or so. For doctors based in rural practice areas, the relevant list size is 350.

Minimum cost

A grant application can only be considered when the total cost of the proposed improvements reaches a specified minimum. The amount is usually reviewed every April (for example, in 1998/99 the threshold was £727 + VAT). If you applied for an improvement grant and the total costs were £500, you would not be eligible for support on minimum cost grounds.

Smaller improvements like this would need to be funded by the practice and counted as a practice expense. You should consult your accountant to establish whether smaller value improvements can be included for tax relief purposes.

The minimum amount is shown in Schedule 2 (point 1) of paragraph 56, assuming your SFA is fully up to date. You should contact your HA or check the financial medical press for the latest allowances.

Eligible works

Existing premises

Only certain types of improvement qualify for acceptance under the scheme. The work must be the improvement of what exists, rather than the provision of new premises. Thus, practices building new accommodation on a greenfield site would not be eligible for a grant. Therefore, premises to be improved would normally be in use already and accepted under the rent and rates scheme (*see* p.3).

Premises not previously used for practice purposes

Newly acquired premises *may* be considered for a grant where the building is deemed by the HA to be suitable for use without alteration and could be accepted under the rent and rates scheme. Clearly, practices contemplating moving into a new building must liaise with their HA to establish whether a grant is payable.

Where this is the case, the grant is subject to financial limits according to the number of practitioners. For the current amounts, you should check Schedule 2 (point 2) of paragraph 56. For 1998/99 the grant payable was £6649 + VAT per doctor, with an overall limit of £23 226).

Significant improvement

The HA must be satisfied that the work is designed to produce significant improvement in the existing practice arrangements for the provision of general medical services. Grants are not designed to help finance repairs or maintenance, which remain the responsibility of the practice. Rather, the scheme is designed to encourage alterations or additions which lead to a benefit for patients or services and comply with minimum standards. The provision of a room for minor surgery or improving wheelchair facilities would qualify for example, whereas redecorating the surgery would be regarded as 'maintenance' and, as such, a practice expense.

Types of eligible work

Examples given in the *Red Book* include:

- the provision of additional rooms (e.g. a consulting room, a minor surgery room or accommodation for attached staff, such as a health visitor). This can be achieved by new building or bringing into practice use rooms not previously used for practice purposes

- enlargement of existing rooms

- improved access (e.g. wheelchair ramp)

- addition to or improvement of toilet and washing facilities (e.g. disabled WC)

- improved lighting, ventilation and heating installations (e.g. replacing old heating system with central heating)

- reasonable extension to telephone facilities (except for a GP registrar when the cost is reimbursable under the GP registrar scheme)

- provision of car and pram parking accommodation

- double glazing

- security systems

- carrying out work required by statute for fire precautions.

Types of work ineligible for a grant

Again, examples from the *Red Book* include:

- the initial provision of premises (new build), including the cost of acquiring land, existing buildings or new buildings

- the initial provision or replacement of furniture, furnishings, floor coverings or equipment (thus, items like desks, chairs, rugs, autoclaves and so on do not qualify for grant)

- repair or maintenance of premises, furniture, furnishings, floor covering or equipment (repairs to a leaking roof, for example)

- restoration of structural damage or deterioration

- any work connected with residential or domestic accommodation

- any work entered into without prior consent from the HA (even if otherwise acceptable). For example, providing wheelchair access prior to formal approval will be ineligible for support. (*Always obtain written approval first*)

- any extension which is not attached to the main building by at least a covered passageway

- that part of any extensions where the total accommodation after the additional accommodation has been completed results in a gross area exceeding the allowances shown in the cost rent schedule in paragraph 51

- any expenses on which a tax allowance is being claimed.

Consult your HA at an early stage to establish what will be acceptable and likely to receive support, and what will not. Priorities may vary and certain types of work receive funding ahead of others. Remember, like cost rent, grant payments are cash-limited and HAs must carefully consider bids against their cash allocation for the year.

The HA may also offer advice or suggestions about other improvements which might be suitable. For example, if you are considering making improvements to surgery security, the HA may provide advice about measures undertaken elsewhere which may be of interest, or recommend a visit by the local crime prevention officer for further advice.

Security of tenure and guarantee of continued use

Doctors will need to demonstrate reasonable security of tenure. Before a grant is paid, doctors are required to sign an agreement form undertaking that the premises for which a grant has been approved will remain in NHS use for a specified minimum period. The period will depend on the value of the grant (shown in

Schedule 2, point 3 of the SFA). For 1998/99 the periods were defined as follows:

- projects with a value up to £19 857 + VAT = 3 years
- projects with a value over £19 857 + VAT = 4 years.

If the practice does not comply with the undertaking, the doctors will have to repay a due proportion, if required to do so by the HA. For example, if a practice receives a grant of £30 000 but after two years ceases to offer NHS services, the HA may require repayment of £15 000 (being half of the original grant because only half of the period of guaranteed use was met).

Consequently, security of tenure must be demonstrated which covers at least the period of guaranteed continued use. That is, the premises should be owned by the practice or held on a lease with an unexpired period of three or four years as appropriate.

Although this describes the regulatory conditions, you can expect the HA to seek longer security of tenure to justify the public investment being made, particularly for larger grants.

NHS use

Grants will only be paid in respect of GMS accommodation. Where premises are not used solely for NHS purposes, the grant will exclude costs associated with non-NHS use and apportion costs for shared improvements, e.g. a common entrance shared by the practice and residential occupiers.

How to apply for an improvement grant

First, consult your HA about any proposals you are considering. Obtaining advice at an early stage can sometimes save you abortive design work and unnecessary expenditure.

When you are ready to proceed, obtain an application form from the HA. This should be completed and returned to the HA together with the following documents:

- sketch plans of premises as they are at present (showing the layout and use of rooms)
- sketch plans of the proposed work
- schedule or specification of works, including the proposed timescale for payment of grant
- estimate of total costs, including fees and VAT, prepared by a builder, architect, surveyor or other suitably qualified person
- copies of any relevant approvals necessary from the local authority to confirm that there are no obstacles to the proposed scheme (e.g. planning permission)
- if the property is held on a lease, the landlord's written consent to the alterations required
- any other documentation specified by your HA in relation to your project.

For smaller projects it may not be necessary for sketch drawings, for example, if you are extending your telephone system, but discuss this first with the HA. Similarly, improving the telephone system will not require planning permission.

Where the cost of the project exceeds a certain amount, the plans, estimates and schedule of works must be produced by an architect, surveyor or other suitably qualified person. The amount is shown at Schedule 2 (point 4). For 1998/99 this was £6649 + VAT.

The HA will then decide whether the application is eligible and can be supported. This will reflect the priority accorded to the proposed works within the HA's premises programme. The HA will inform the practice whether the application has been approved (either formally or in principle) and the proportion of grant support available. The HA has discretion to offer between 33% and 66% and the amount offered will depend on local policy and availability of funds. The HA will also indicate whether any conditions apply in respect of the target date for payment of the grant. If the decision is not to your satisfaction, you should discuss the circumstances with the HA. It may be possible to submit more arguments in favour of your application or to modify it in some way.

If you intend to proceed, the HA will normally want to see three competitive tenders or estimates for the works proposed, if these have not already been provided. The grant will be based on the lowest of the three tenders, although the practice is free to use the contractor of their choice. There may be some exceptional circumstances when the HA is prepared to accept fewer than three tenders, but this will need to be agreed beforehand.

With tenders received, the HA will give formal approval and issue an agreement form enabling you to proceed. This will set out the amount of grant to be paid on completion of the works (or to be paid in instalments during the course of the work) and the period for which the premises are to continue in NHS use. No grant, or instalment of grant, can be paid until the agreement form has been completed and signed by the doctors.

Payments

Where the estimated cost of the project is greater than the amount shown in paragraph 56, Schedule 2.5 (£6649 + VAT in 1998/99), the practice may request payment of the grant in instalments. The grant can then be paid in stages up to 90% of the total amount committed. For each instalment you will need to submit appropriate receipts, architect's certificates, etc., stating the total costs incurred to date. The balance will not be paid until all the final documentation has been received. The instalment payments will be the appropriate proportion (i.e. 33% to 66%) of the approved cost incurred. Where the estimated costs are below the amount above, or instalments are not requested, the grant will be payable at the completion of the project.

When the work is finished and all the payments made, a final claim needs to be made on a form supplied by the HA. This form should be accompanied by all receipted bills and certificates as appropriate. The grant (or balance of grant) can then be paid, although the HA will probably wish to inspect the premises beforehand.

What if the project costs or timescale overrun?

Any variation from the agreed plan must be notified to the HA as soon as possible. Clearly, increases in costs must be discussed as there is no obligation or guarantee that the HA will increase the grant payment. Delays in the completion of the project can significantly affect the HA's ability to pay the grant if, for example, it shifts from one financial year to another. It is in your interests, therefore, to try to plan and manage the project well, and to inform the HA immediately any variations become apparent.

Tax implications

Practitioners should note that the cost of work cannot qualify for both improvement grant and tax relief. The claim form includes a declaration to state that no part of the cost on which a grant has been claimed will be included in tax relief claims.

In practice, it is unusual for tax relief to be given on the types of item eligible for improvement grant and the proportion of grant available (33% to 66%) compares well to the current tax relief arrangements. So it is often the case that a grant is more advantageous.

You should always seek professional advice from your accountant as to whether it would be more favourable to claim tax relief or an improvement grant.

Can grants be combined with cost rents?

Subject to the agreement of your HA, it is possible to combine a grant with a cost rent scheme, where the cost rent project involves modification of an existing building or modification of an acquired building. Where a grant is approved, the amount is then deducted from the cost rent limit. An example is given in Box 1.3 to illustrate the effects of a grant combined with cost rent.

Although the cost rent limit is reduced, the advantage to the practice is that the grant reduces the amount of capital to be borrowed. For owner-occupiers this should hasten the point where the current market rent (notional rent) exceeds cost rent.

Can doctors appeal against improvement grant decisions?

Where you are dissatisfied with the decision of the HA concerning

---

Box 1.3:   Combining a grant with a cost rent scheme

Cost rent limit	=	£350 000
Reimbursement pa (assumes percentage of 10%)	=	£35 000

With grant of £50 000:

Cost rent limit	=	£350 000 *minus* £50 000
		= £300 000

---

an improvement grant application or claim, representations can be made in writing to the Secretary of State within two months of the date of notification by the HA of its decision.

The private sector

So far, this chapter has reviewed the SFA tools available to assist practices in the improvement or development of premises, and the role the HA has to play. The examples given have generally followed GP-led schemes, whereby practices take responsibility for the development of new premises or improvement of existing surgeries.

But there are other players in the marketplace who may be able to provide surgery premises on doctors' behalf. This section is a very brief introduction to the potential options for the involvement of the private sector. Once again, your HA is a good source of advice, knowledge and expertise in guiding you through the benefits and disadvantages of working with the private sector.

Private finance initiative (PFI) and public/private partnerships (PPP)

It has become an accepted part of government policy to explore and encourage the involvement of the private sector in the provision of primary care facilities, where this is appropriate and provides value for money. Partnerships with the private sector can produce successful outcomes and sometimes may be the most appropriate, indeed only, option for achieving change.

The PFI placed increased emphasis on the potential and future role of the private sector in all public sector developments and private finance is being encouraged in the NHS where its use represents good value for money.

There has been much debate on the value of the PFI and current policy continues to highlight the potential role of increased partnerships with the private sector. It is fair to say that much of the PFI debate has focused on larger, multi-million pound projects such as hospital developments, whereas private sector involvement at primary care level has been more limited.

In many ways, the cost rent scheme can be regarded as an example of the use of private finance in the primary care sector, in that doctors are responsible for raising the capital through banks and financial institutions, rather than using public capital to develop surgeries. However, cost rent schemes are still generally GP-led and GP-owned.

But the market for private sector involvement in the GP field has matured, with more companies and developers willing to invest in and own GP premises, with a better understanding of GP premises issues, and a recognition of the opportunities and constraints which that brings.

When considering options for development therefore, you should be aware that a private partnership scheme may be suitable with mutual benefits to the parties concerned.

Examples

There are a number of companies that are willing to develop purpose-built premises to an agreed specification, with an agreement to lease those premises once completed, provided it is financially viable. It should be remembered that doctors represent 'blue-chip tenants' for the private sector and a surgery development is a good long-term investment for a developer or subsequent buyer. For the doctors, the objective is to obtain the use of a high-quality surgery which meets their needs, under a suitable lease and at an affordable market rent. From the developer's perspective, they are seeking a cost-effective investment with good tenants under a suitable lease.

One of the keys to success will be effective negotiation with the private party to ensure that the best deal possible is obtained. For example, many developers may seek a lease of 21 years or more, but it does not follow that this would be the most convenient position for the practice and this should be negotiable. The HA can provide you with help and advice, or refer you to other professionals to assist you.

A project need not necessarily involve an obvious private partner such as a development company. The third party could be a local housing association which agrees to incorporate primary care facilities as part of a larger housing development. It can be advantageous to a private developer or housing association to include a surgery as part of a wider scheme if this provides assistance in obtaining planning permission ('planning gain').

There are some companies which will also consider buying existing surgery premises from a practice for subsequent leasing, which could include further improvement to the surgery.

Why choose a private-led approach?

In some circumstances, there are very limited options for a new development because of a lack of sites in a particular area. Buildings or sites may only become available via a private party who wishes to act as the developer/owner of any scheme. In other circumstances, a careful appraisal of the options may identify a third-party scheme as the most effective means of achieving your premises needs.

It may also be a preference of the practice, where the partners do not wish to be owner-occupiers and responsible for a large loan, but prefer instead to be tenants in a leased building.

Where cash-limited resources are already fully committed, the private partnership route may offer a suitable option funded via market rent.

Can the private sector approach really work?

Fortunately, the answer to this is yes, although not in every circumstance. As with a GP-led approach, close liaison with the HA, good preparation, option appraisal and sound professional advice are important components in considering a private sector scheme.

There is no scope here to explore the many variations that may be possible and the range of factors to be considered when contemplating a private sector scheme or before entering into an agreement. Factors governing a successful outcome include agreement to design, layout and specification, satisfactory lease arrangements, agreed rental values, timescales, business case approval from the Regional Office in some cases and so on.

The HA may have experience of particular companies or developers and recommend those with a good track record and understanding of GP premises matters. (Equally, they may advise you of potential problems with some companies.)

Sound legal advice is absolutely crucial if a third-party scheme is to be successful. Because a lease will be involved, experienced legal advice is required to produce terms and conditions which best protect the practice's interest before entering into a legally binding agreement.

In the writer's view, there is no single recommended route for creating high-quality surgery facilities. Doctors need to consider the various options and their particular circumstances before reaching a judgement, working in close liaison with their HA to establish what is feasible.

In some circumstances this may mean a partnership with a private party or non-NHS body, and in others a GP-led approach is more desirable and appropriate. Either way, it is necessary to keep your HA on board and to maximise the support and expertise that may be available. A practice's desire to have improved premises is often shared by the HA and it is therefore in everybody's interest to adopt an open, collaborative approach.

Can the private sector attract and retain

2

The designer's and project manager's viewpoint

NEIL NIBLETT

Procedures

Initial health authority approval

A doctor must have health authority (HA) approval to build new premises. Several factors can affect their decision, for example, present premises and patient list size; but now, more importantly, HA budgets.

Each project will need to be included in a financial year's budget. Each application should now include:

- estimate of cost, including any abnormal site conditions
- anticipated completion date
- sketch if available
- site location if available.

The procedures for 'new build' are slightly different from that for extension developments. It may be possible to obtain up to 66%

grant aid from the HA. Reference to your general manager is recommended.

Do not proceed until you have HA approval.

Land

If you are looking for a site, remember the following:

- check that the site itself is not affected by culverts, high voltage cables, gas mains, coal mines, and so on – whilst the site may be ideally located, it may be expensive to develop
- the HA must approve the location and the value, subject to the district valuer's (DV) assessment
- it is essential to obtain planning permission and a site investigation before committing yourself to purchase.

Site investigation

This should be carried out to ascertain ground conditions.

Sketch scheme

The surgery design must be in accordance with the general notes issued by the HA and the cost rent scheme. Floor areas should be shown in schedules. Patient flow and confidentiality must be considered.

The surgery will also need to comply with the Disabled Persons Act and Disability Discrimination Act for both patients and staff.

The NHS Estates has produced Health Building Note 46, which may prove useful.

HA approval

The design, when agreed by the client, must be submitted to the HA, who may consult the medical advisor. They approve, in principle, the scheme in terms of the floor areas, room sizes and general layout.

The introduction of new cost rent schedules from 1 November 1997 means that a medical practice must justify *all* the space they propose to create.

The HA will pay particular attention to the supervision of patients, storage of medical records and confidentiality at the reception area.

Provision for carrying out minor surgery should be considered, also provision of other primary healthcare team members.

Budgets

Following HA approval, budget costs must be prepared and submitted to the HA. These are to show the building costs, fixtures and any abnormal site costs to be claimed. The HA will then produce an interim cost rent assessment.

Funding approval

You will require funding for the project. A number of high street banks and the General Practice Finance Corporation (GPFC), a funding arm of Norwich Union, have considerable experience in lending for GP premises. It may be necessary to obtain an interim loan from a high street bank before looking into a fixed rate with the GPFC. Commercial organisations and insurance companies may seem cheap, but usually are not.

The GPFC is also now offering very good finance deals, in particular fixed loans over 25 years. This rate alters daily and it is of paramount importance that careful negotiation on timing of the loan is considered.

The best advice is for you to consult your accountant, who should be able to arrange 100% funding of the project over 20–25 years at a competitive rate. However, no two cases are the same.

Planning permission

Detailed planning permission will be needed for the banks to confirm a loan. This can be done using the sketch scheme drawings previously prepared for the HA. At this stage you would not yet have involved yourself in expensive fees. Typical architectural fees which you should expect to have to pay are indicated on p.111. Other consultants' fees would be extra.

Working drawings, building regulation approval and specification

Before commencing with this stage you must be sure you want to proceed. At this point, large architectural fees can be expected.

Full and detailed discussions are necessary to clarify design and specification. It is essential that you cover every aspect of the project.

Tenders

In accordance with the HA guidelines, three tenders are to be invited. You are not obliged to accept the lowest, but the HA will base their cost rent on the lowest tender.

Ensure that the drawings and specifications are suitable for competitive tendering. On receipt of tenders, ensure that all contractors have included all that is necessary to complete the building. If in doubt, *ask*.

Full HA approval

All information should be submitted to the HA for their approval before signing a building contract. Check with the HA what items are allowable under the cost rent scheme.

Health and safety

It is now necessary to appoint a planning supervisor under the Construction (Design and Management) Regulations 1994. This *must* be done. Usually the architect will carry out the role. Usual fees are between 0.5% and 2% of the construction cost. The fee for this service is now included within the professional fee allowance contained in the cost rent schedules.

Contract documentation

On every project a form of contract is required. The joint contracts tribunal offers standard forms of building agreements.

Ensure that you are aware of what you are signing. Have all the relevant clauses explained. Do not sign until you own the land and you have funding arranged. A set of documents must be signed, they consist of:

- all the drawings
- the specification/bill of quantities
- the submitted tender
- the contract.

VAT

VAT is payable on the building costs and professional fees at the prevailing rate. VAT may be charged on the land. Reference to your legal advisor and accountant is essential.

Supervision

As works proceed, advise the HA of any change or variations immediately; they may well approve abnormal costs if problems are encountered. However, beware. Exceptional site costs are those that are foreseeable.

Interim cost rent submission

As soon as the building is finished, a practice completion certificate should be issued. From the date of the certificate, cost rent is paid.

This certificate, together with the last valuation and a receipted account of monies received to date from the contractor, should be submitted immediately to the HA.

Final account

Upon certification of the final account, all receipts should be submitted to the HA to enable them to calculate the final cost rent payment.

Appointment of design team

When considering a development it is essential to obtain good and correct advice, particularly as healthcare projects, whilst straightforward in engineering terms, can be complicated in project management. By obtaining the best advice and following the correct procedures, dangers can be avoided and thus the project becomes a total design and affordable success.

Most projects will require the following professional guidance:

- architectural
- building cost control
- planning supervision
- structural appraisal.

It is possible that further guidance may be required on land availability and party wall involvement.

Consider your design team carefully. They need to be experienced in primary healthcare projects and understand NHS guidance and HA procedures, as well as possessing a knowledge of legal and financial issues.

Land search

Consider very carefully potential sites for development and obtain advice on site conditions, services, etc. Try and obtain the DV's assessment of the site value.

If you are acquiring a new site have a site investigation carried out and, if possible, obtain at least outline planning permission before you commit yourself to a purchase. If you can obtain detail planning, so much the better.

Design

- Surgery design is very important. The building must function correctly and comply with the latest NHS guidance. Health Building Note 46 and the cost rent commentary are useful reference points, and are available from the NHS Executive in Leeds.
- The surgery must also comply with the latest disabled requirements as defined by the Building Regulations and the Disability Discrimination Act.
- Patient flow, control and confidentiality are all important ingredients for a successful design.
- Quality construction also provides for a quality building requiring low maintenance and low running costs.
- The HA must approve the design. Every square metre must be justified. The HA will pay particular attention to supervision of patients, storage of medical records and confidentiality at reception, as well as the number, type and size of clinical and administration rooms.
- The NHS Executive is keen to promote quality buildings and hence well-designed buildings will be encouraged. Good design need not be an expensive design.

Costings

The design team will prepare cost budgets as the scheme progresses – you should ensure you understand these budgets. There are also strict limits for premises under the cost rent scheme and these should also be understood.

At the time of considering a new site, make the HA aware of any abnormal site conditions or stringent planning requirements. These may well add to the cost of the project, but may also be included for exceptional site costs under the cost rent scheme. **Remember**, if you are developing under the notional rent method, there is no facility for exceptional site costs.

Planning, detailed design, tender process

- As the project progresses the design team will deal with all matters relating to the detailed design and approval process.
- It is important that you understand each stage and *communicate* with the team.
- *Do not* be afraid to question design changes, costings or the programme.
- *Ensure* you understand the tender process and the contract documentation.
- Allow the design team to manage the project smoothly.
- *Do not* get involved in contractual negotiations.
- *Ensure* the HA is advised of each stage and that the correct information is issued to them at the appropriate stages.
- You must advise the HA of any changes to the plans.

Surgery design criteria

- Surgery design is essentially a *functional elemental building*, which means if it does not function it does not work!
- Patient flow, control and confidentiality are vital elements in the design process.
- The need for users of the building to access all parts freely provides for efficient use of time throughout the day.
- There are two basic concepts to surgery design: the 'cruciform' and the 'doughnut'. Both have advantages and disadvantages.

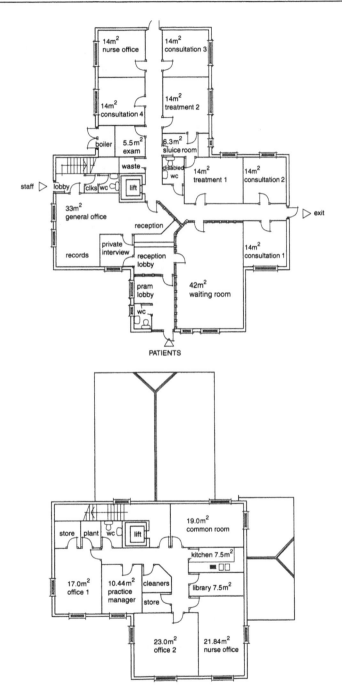

Figure 2.1 Surgery design: the cruciform.

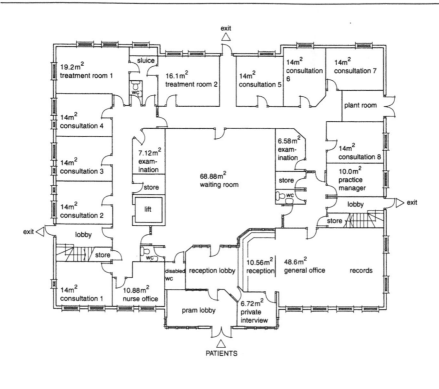

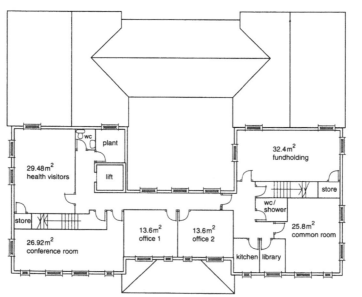

Figure 2.2 Surgery design: the doughnut.

Cruciform (Figure 2.1)

- This provides for a building that has good patient control and easy access to all areas.
- It maximises external wall space to provide natural light and ventilation to all rooms.
- It also provides for interesting elevational treatment.
- Its disadvantages are cost. It is not economic in building cost terms, as it has a high wall to floor ratio.

Doughnut (Figure 2.2)

- This provides for a tighter shape usually arranged around a central waiting area servicing the clinical rooms.
- The advantages are that patient flow to the clinic area is quicker, building costs are more efficient and the site area required is reduced.
- The disadvantages are that the actual circular space is larger and thus expensive; or if corridors are reduced or omitted then communication with the administration area is restricted.

It is essential that a correct and detailed design brief is discussed and established with the design team.

The final outcome is dependent upon GP input and design team experience. Together they can, subject to site conditions, produce a quality building that will satisfy the requirements of the GPs, users and HAs for the foreseeable future.

Schedule of architectural services

5%	Stage A: feasibility study	Analyse the site and undertake preliminary discussions with the local planning authority. Obtain service enquiries from statutory undertakings. Take client's brief and prepare a basic sketch scheme to ensure that the project is viable.

continued

10%	Stage B: outline proposals	Carry out a detailed survey of the site. Prepare further sketch schemes and submit for HA comments.
20%	Stage C: scheme design	Develop the scheme design, taking into account the client's and HA's comments, and prepare scheme design drawings. Apply for local authority planning permission.
25%	Stage D: detailed design	Prepare detailed design drawings, submit for building regulation approval and obtain fire officer's comments. Co-ordinate the work of any subcontractors, suppliers or consultants.
20%	Stage E: production information	Prepare production information in the form of specifications/bills of quantities, schedules and further drawings. Submit to the HA for their approval.
5%	Stage F: tenders	Prepare a list of contractors and invite firm price tenders and advise on the appointment of a contractor. Submit tenders to the HA. Amend cost budget and programme as necessary.
5%	Stage G: project planning	Ensure that all necessary approvals are obtained. Prepare contract documents and arrange for their signing.
5%	Stage H: operations on site	Visit the site as appropriate to inspect generally the progress and quality of work. Issue valuation certificates and administer the terms of the contract. Make periodic financial reports to the client.
5%	Stage I: completion	Administer the terms of the contract through to completion. Advise on the contractor's final account. Submit accounts to the HA for interim and final cost rent assessment.

The do's and don'ts of controlling your architect: a guide to GPs embarking on a new surgery development or refurbishing existing premises

If embarking on a cost rent scheme or improvement grant, consideration must always be given to very careful budget control, and professional expertise in this field is most important.

It is frequently found that doctors have, for many reasons, been somewhat dissatisfied with their new surgery premises. Upon analysing the complaint, it is found that it is lack of communication and understanding between client and architect that causes problems. We intend, therefore, to run through a typical surgery project, highlighting the *do's* and *don'ts* of controlling your architect.

These points should always be asked and considered:

- *Do* go for an architectural practice with experience of surgery design and an understanding of the *Red Book*.

- *Do* go for commercial firms of architects. Ask about fees, timescales, workloads and so on, staffing levels and commitments.

- *Do* ensure that the firm has valid and adequate professional indemnity insurance.

Fees

- *Do* ask about fees. There is a recommended fee scale, but check what service it relates to and whether expenses are inclusive or exclusive.
- *Do* obtain a written quotation on fees and expenses.
- *Do* obtain a breakdown of fees in relation to each work stage – thus, if a project fails, fees can easily be calculated.

Services

Do ask what service is to be provided. Other services could be extra, for example:

- surveys, model making, perspectives
- interior design, cost planning
- town planning appeals, project management
- site supervision.

Consultants

- *Do* check if any other consultants are required or proposed, for example:
  - quantity surveyor
  - mechanical and electrical engineer
  - structural engineer
  - landscape consultant
  - planning consultant
  - land surveyor
  - geologist
  - valuer
  - estate agent
  - interior designer.
- *Do* obtain fees and written quotations – checking expenses.
- *Do* make sure you understand each consultant's role and how fees are calculated.
- *Do not* engage any consultant until you are in receipt of formal HA approval.

Land

- *Do* agree some professional advice prior to the purchase of the site. You need to check:

- ground stability, soil analysis, service enquiries (e.g. gas, water, electricity, etc.)

- planning requirements.

• *Do* have a fixed-fee feasibility study carried out. This should show whether or not the scheme is potentially viable. Ask for budget costings and refer back to your initial costing plan.

HA approval

• *Do* get the architect to prepare sketch schemes of your proposal.

• *Do not* accept a scheme if not totally to your approval. Consider the possible need for an extension in the future – can this easily be achieved?

• Ensure that the floor areas are in line with the *Red Book* requirements.

• Upon agreement of a scheme, submit to the HA.

• *Do not* engage your architect to produce any further information until you are in receipt of formal HA approval.

Scheme design

• Upon approval from the HA, a full detailed brief should be taken.

• *Do* make sure you emphasize your needs to the architect.

• *Do* make sure the architect understands your cost budget.

• *Do* make sure the architect and quantity surveyor produce a further cost plan and estimate of building costs.

• *Do* obtain a programme of work envisaged by the architect – your HA will also require this.

• *Do not* proceed past this stage until in receipt of planning permission and full knowledge of land purchase.

Detailed design

- Be careful of the choice of materials.

- *Do not* accept materials or design amendments until the cost implications are carefully considered.

Production information

- *Do* be sure you understand the specification, from foundations to the finished building, even down to the last nut and bolt.

- It is advisable to nominate one of your partners to deal with the detailing aspects and be in direct liaison with the architect.

Tenders

- *Do not* get involved with the seeking of tenders. By all means give a list of preferred contractors to the architect, but let him or her check their credibility and seek tenders.

- *Do not* accept a tender if over budget, ask the quantity surveyor to produce a list of items that can be cut back.

3

The solicitor's viewpoint

LYNNE ABBESS

Introduction

The opportunity to invest in 'new' surgery premises should be an
asset in every sense of the word. However, unless you put
yourselves in the best position to 'get it right' you could find
instead that your asset has turned into a huge liability.

Within this chapter you will find the issues you are most likely to
face in conjunction with the development of a greenfield site or the
'substantial modification' of a property which is either bought for
the purposes of conversion or which is already owned. It should be
appreciated, however, that inevitably it is not possible to deal with
each and every situation, or to provide a foolproof solution to
every problem, as each case must be dealt with on its facts. Indeed,
it would be most unwise to assume that the basic principles
discussed here may be relied upon in each and every case.

Undoubtedly, it is essential for appropriate specialist professional
advice to be sought from a very early stage before embarking upon

such a scheme. Furthermore, that advice should be taken from an expert professional in each of their appropriate fields. You should not assume that the complex rules and regulations surrounding NHS GPs' practice life or the construction details of surgery premises are familiar to every professional in the country, and the last thing you would want to find is that you are being treated as a guinea pig. *Your* scheme is likely to be the largest investment you make in your professional (and possibly your domestic) life and you should ensure that you put yourself in the best possible position to receive proper advice from the outset in order to enable you to structure not only the scheme itself, but also the impact upon your partnership, in the most satisfactory way. It is never easy, and may be impossible, to rewrite history after the event, particularly if the circumstances in which it becomes necessary arise as a result of a dispute.

Furthermore, anyone who even contemplates entering into the commitment of taking on new surgery premises (whether they be owned or leased) without an up-to-date partnership agreement catering for the situation is asking for trouble! The very fact that a partnership can be dissolved at will upon a moment's notice, without the need to give reasons, would leave the property owners – and indeed the non-property owners in occupation of the surgery premises – in a seriously exposed position.

The advice in this chapter will hopefully enable you to avoid falling into some of the more obvious traps.

Basic principles of property law

It is difficult adequately to explain the points you need to consider without first considering the basic principles relating to property ownership and occupation. The application of simple common sense is not sufficient because, like an iceberg, the majority of the problems lie beneath the surface and are not immediately apparent to the lay person. Accordingly, the following pages attempt to set out a very basic guide to property ownership and occupation and to identify some of the hidden traps.

Ownership

'Ownership' relates either to a freehold or to a long lease at a 'peppercorn' or nominal ground rent. (This can be contrasted with a short lease – typically anything from six months to 25 years – during which a current market rent is payable throughout each year of the term.)

It is necessary to distinguish between the legal title to a property (which is held on trust), as evidenced by the names on the title deeds to the property (the trustees), and the equitable or beneficial title, which lurks behind the scenes (and which represents what would normally be regarded as the 'actual ownership' of the property) (Figure 3.1).

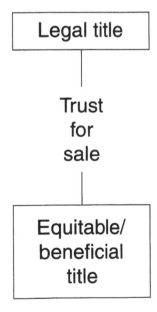

Ownership of property

(Freehold or Leasehold)

Figure 3.1 Legal and equitable interest.

Legal interest

The legal title will usually be evidenced through a land certificate (where there is no mortgage) or a charge certificate (which identifies not only the owner of the land but also the mortgagee, i.e. the lender). As the whole of England and Wales is now subject to compulsory registration, there are increasingly fewer examples of unregistered land.

Equitable interest

A sole owner will have both the legal and equitable interests in the property vested in his or her name (Figure 3.2a). In the case of joint

Ownership of property

(Freehold or Leasehold)

Sole owner:

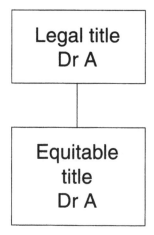

Figure 3.2a Sole ownership.

Ownership of property

(Freehold or Leasehold)

Joint owners:

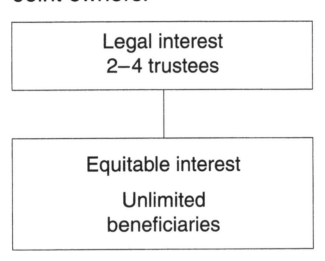

> Legal interest
> 2–4 trustees

> Equitable interest
>
> Unlimited
> beneficiaries

1 Legal title: minimum of two and maximum of four trustees.

2 For example, of five owning doctors:
   Legal title: Drs A B C + D upon trust for
   Equitable title: Drs A B C D + E

Figure 3.2b Joint ownership.

ownership, no matter how many equitable owners there may be, a maximum of only four names are permitted on the legal title (i.e. the title deeds) to the property. These owners are said to hold the property 'upon trust' for the equitable owners (Figure 3.2b). Thus in a case where there are, for example, five equitable owners, it would be common practice to find the names of Doctors A, B, C and D appearing on the legal title to the property, who would be expressed to hold the property 'upon trust' for Doctors A, B, C, D and E. Alternatively, it may be considered appropriate for only Doctors A and B, for example, to hold the legal title upon trust for all five owners. In such circumstances, it is apparent that the position of Dr E will need to be protected as his/her name will not appear on the face of the title deeds as evidence of his/her ownership.

Legal interest: joint tenants

Trustees will always hold the legal title as joint tenants (Figure 3.3). The legal maxim of *ius accrescendi* applies, whereby there is no subdivision of ownership between the joint tenants, and in the event of the death of one of them, the remaining joint tenants will automatically inherit the share of the deceased owner.

Equitable interest: joint tenants or tenants in common

This may be owned either as a joint tenancy (as above) or as a tenancy in common, which is more usual within a business arrangement such as a partnership. Under a tenancy in common, each owner holds a distinct share of the property. This may be in equal or unequal shares, such as in the case of four owners; they could each hold a 25% share or they could hold in shares of, for example, 40%, 30%, 20%, 10%. If one of the joint owners were to die, his/her share would pass to his/her estate to be distributed in accordance with the terms of his/her will. For this reason it can be understood that it is essential that in the case of the joint ownership of partnership property, proper provision is made within the context of a partnership agreement to deal with the share of a partner in the event of retirement or death.

Leasehold interest

Where there is a lease (whether in circumstances of a long lease with a capital value or a short lease where a current market rent is

Ownership of property

(Freehold or Leasehold)

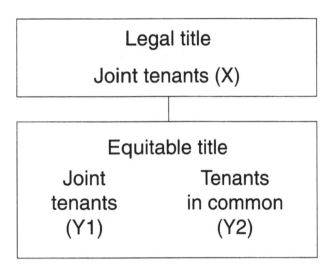

For example, X holds the property for Y1 as joint tenants on a trust for sale.

X holds the property for Y2 as joint tenants on a trust for sale and as tenants in common [in equal shares/in the following shares:

Dr A – 50%
Dr B – 25%
Dr C – 25%]

Figure 3.3 Joint tenancy / tenancy in common.

payable on an annual basis), a contractual relationship will exist between the landlord and tenant. Figure 3.4 deals simply with the legal title to the property. The legal title to a lease will be evidenced by two documents:

1   the lease itself, which is produced in two parts – the original lease (signed by the landlord and retained by the tenant) and the counterpart lease (signed by the tenant and retained by the landlord)

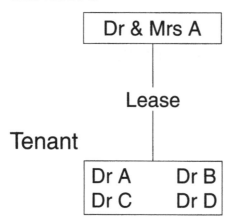

Ownership of property
(Leasehold)

Landlord

Dr & Mrs A

Lease

Tenant

Dr A	Dr B
Dr C	Dr D

Figure 3.4 Leasehold interest.

2   if the lease is for a term of 21 years or more, it will be register-
able at the Land Registry and in addition to the lease documentation, a land or charge certificate will be issued in respect of the
leasehold title (in addition to that issued in respect of the
freehold title as discussed above).

It is stressed, however, that these documents deal only with the
legal interest in the property and not with the equitable interest (for
which see below).

Figure 3.5 marries together the principles we have considered so
far in dealing with both the freehold and leasehold titles and the
legal and equitable interests.

The need to produce evidence in writing documenting the
intention of the parties with regard to their joint ownership, particularly with regard to any party whose name does not appear on
the legal title, has already been mentioned. Two examples follow
which demonstrate what can go wrong where parties have failed to
take the appropriate steps to protect their interests.

Ownership of property
(Leasehold)

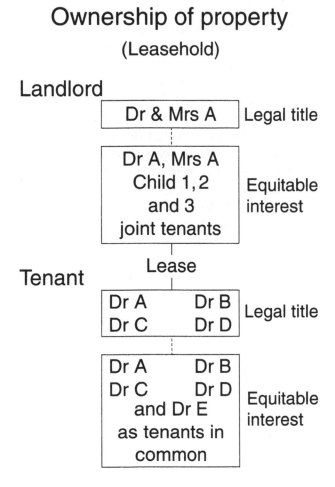

Figure 3.5 Freehold/ leasehold interest: legal/ equitable title.

Example 1

Doctors A and B joined together in partnership at a time when Dr A was on the verge of entering into a cost rent scheme. It was always the intention that the partners would purchase the property and enter into the scheme jointly. Indeed, all the costs associated with the acquisition and development of the property, the shortfall on the mortgage repayments (as the cost rent reimbursement did not meet the mortgage outgoings in full) and the premiums payable on the collateral life policy effected on the life of Dr A, were paid by the parties in 50/50 shares. Some time later, as a result of a dispute, Dr A claimed that he was the sole owner of the property. Much to Dr B's surprise, he discovered that regardless of the fact that he had been meeting half the costs of the property, his name was not on the legal title documents.

Dr A expressed surprise when Dr B claimed half the value of the property. As a result of this, Dr B was forced to issue proceedings for a declaration of the High Court that he was indeed entitled to a 50% equitable interest. Some four years after the issue of proceedings the matter was eventually settled out of court and Dr B was entitled to recoup 50% of his share of the equity in the property together with a large part (although not all) of his costs. However, had there been a properly drawn partnership agreement declaring that the parties held the equitable interest of the property in equal shares, it would not have been in Dr A's interest to seek to resist the claim as he would not have had a leg to stand on.

Example 2

Doctors A and B jointly owned a property which was subject to a General Practice Finance Corporation (GPFC) mortgage. They received notional rent in respect of their ownership of the property, the mortgage outgoings being deducted at source by the health authority (HA). The balance of notional rent was paid into the partnership and over a period of time this sum increased to a level considerably in excess of the mortgage outgoings following a series of reviews.

During the course of this period, a new partner, Dr C, joined the partnership. He expressly declined to purchase a share of the property and he was permitted to occupy as a licensee (see below). However, once again nothing was documented in writing.

Several years later there followed a dispute with Dr C, who, much to the surprise of Drs A and B, declared that he held a one-third equitable interest in the property. Dr C's name did not appear on the legal title to the property, nor was he known to the GPFC. However, Dr C issued proceedings in support of his claim, citing in support of his argument that as the partnership accounts had shown him to be entitled to receive one-third of the notional rent, this was evidence of the intention of the parties that he should be a one-third owner of the property.

Whilst it was evident that Dr C had not at any time bought into the property, after a number of years of litigation, Drs A and B decided to 'pay off' Dr C in order to bring the litigation to an end, and accordingly a lump sum payment was made to him. However, had there been a proper partnership agreement in existence, declaring that the property was intended to be owned by Drs A and B only, and declaring Dr C's position as a licensee, it would not have been worth Dr C's while pursuing the claim and Drs A and B would have been saved the settlement payment and the costs, not to mention the time and hassle, of enduring several years of litigation.

The moral from these two stories is evident. If you wish to avoid the prospect of litigation, you must get your house in order, which means entering into a proper declaration of trust setting down the parties' intention with regard to the ownership, shareholding and occupation of the property; this can usually be incorporated within a partnership agreement.

Occupation

There is no greater right on the part of an individual to enter and occupy privately owned surgery premises than to do so in your own home. Figure 3.6 demonstrates the range of categories of occupation, to include unlawful occupation (trespassing). As has been evident in the case of equitable ownership, there are also hidden traps in the case of occupation of property, as deemed rights may be acquired unless the owner takes steps to prevent such rights from arising.

Owner occupation

Naturally an owner of a property is, *prima facie*, entitled to occupy that property (unless he or she has already agreed to give exclusive occupation of the property to a third party under a tenancy/lease, for which see below).

Occupation of property

A Owner-occupier
- Sole owner
- Joint owner

B Lessee
- Within Landlord and Tenant Act 1954 Part II
- Outside Landlord and Tenant Act

C Licensee

D Trespasser

Figure 3.6 Bases of occupation.

Tenancy/lease

A lease grants a tenant the lawful right to occupy the property throughout the term granted by the lease. However, a business tenancy may also arise under the Landlord and Tenant Act 1954 Part II without there being any written form of documentation, simply by the owner of property allowing someone to take up occupation and pay rent. This situation should be avoided at all costs because of the rights it carries with it, as set out below. Any basis of occupation of property should be considered carefully *before* occupation is taken up and be recorded in writing. If a lease is to be granted, two alternatives should be considered, as described below.

Tenancy/lease within the Landlord and Tenant Act 1954 Part II

An occupier of property with rights under the 1954 Act may be entitled to continue to occupy that property (i.e. to have security of tenure) *beyond* the term of the lease granted and (where no written documentation was entered into) where the Court construes that it was the intent of the parties to create a tenancy. In such circumstances, it may be difficult for you (as landlord) to evict such a party from your property and if you were to be successful in doing so (by being able to satisfy the Court that you qualify under one of the grounds set down in section 38 of the 1954 Act) you would have to pay the evicted tenant compensation based on a multiple of the rateable value of the property.

The added problem is that even if you have entered into a written document purporting to limit the rights of the individual to occupy your property, the Court may deem that your intention was other than as declared in black and white in the agreement (see below under 'Licence').

The benefit to a tenant of a lease granted within the 1954 Act is that not only does the tenant have the lawful right to occupy the property during the term of the lease but (subject to a few exceptions contained within section 38 as referred to above) s/he has an automatic right to renew the lease at the end of the term on substantially similar terms. This puts the tenant in a far stronger bargaining position at the time of renewal with regard to the negotiation of a whole variety of factors, not least being the reviewed rent.

Tenancy/lease granted outside the 1954 Act

It is possible to enter into a written agreement (and evidence in writing *is* required in these circumstances) and to seek a Court Order under section 38(4) of the 1954 Act whereby the security of tenure provisions granted by the Act are excluded. The effect of this is that the tenant has the lawful right to occupy the property throughout the duration of the term of the lease but has no automatic right to renew upon the expiry of that term.

In practice, the landlord may have no objection to renewing the lease, but the fact that there is no automatic right of renewal puts the tenant in a far weaker negotiating position in seeking to secure his/

her position for the future. Thus, the landlord may demand a higher rent or seek to impose more unreasonable terms than contained in the original lease.

Licence

Alternatively, an owner of property may determine that s/he does not wish to grant a tenancy/lease either within or outside the provisions of the 1954 Act. S/he may, however, be prepared to permit the occupation of his/her property 'for the time being'.

In such circumstances, it is possible to grant a licence, the effect of which is to allow the licensee the lawful right to occupy the property either for a short set period of time (usually less than six months) or 'for the time being' but subject to notice being served to require vacant possession to be given.

If such a relationship is not evidenced in writing, there is a serious risk that in the event of the licensor requiring vacant possession, the licensee may claim to have security of tenure as a tenant under the 1954 Act. There would be no suggestion in such circumstances that the lease would be outside the 1954 Act as there would not be the evidence of a Court Order confirming exclusion.

Even if the relationship is evidenced in writing in a document entitled 'a Licence', the Court has the power to consider whether the parties genuinely intended to enter into the relationship of licensor/licensee or whether there is evidence that some other relationship was intended, that is, it will not necessarily follow the heading of the document. If, for example, the licensee has been asked to pay rent or to contribute to the structural maintenance of the property, this may be construed as evidence that the parties intended a tenancy to be entered into within the 1954 Act, thus giving security of tenure.

If a licence has been created, it may be determined on reasonable notice, which in the case of a professional person would normally be for not less than three months, although it may be possible to extend this further (e.g. to six or nine months) depending upon the circumstances of the case.

Trespasser

A trespasser does not enjoy rights to occupy the property on any basis, even temporarily, and can expect steps to be taken to evict him/her with immediate effect.

Occupation of surgery premises by non-owning GP partners

It is not uncommon to find that the surgery premises are owned by some but not all of the partners and the question of the basis of occupation of the non-partners must be given careful consideration. The law weighs everything up in the balance and the following factors should be taken into consideration:

1   In the case of a lease:
*   the ability of the owners (landlords) to charge rent and to require the non-owners (tenants) to contribute to the maintenance of the fabric and structure of the property

    versus

*   the security of tenure given to the occupier (tenants).

2   In the case of a licence:
*   the requirement for the owners (licensors) to bear the costs of maintenance of the structure and exterior of the property without the right to charge rent

    versus

*   the lack of security for the occupiers (licensees).

It should be acknowledged in any event that the payment of rent in either scenario may not be applicable bearing in mind that the landlord GPs will be receiving the benefit of notional/cost rent from the HA as owners of the property. However, many owning GPs consider it unfair for their non-owning colleagues to be entitled to occupy their property without having to bear any of the costs of maintenance whilst being entitled to enjoy a full share of the profits of the partnership. In order to overcome this dilemma, it may be considered appropriate for the owning GPs as landlords to grant a lease to the partnership as a whole as tenants, imposing upon the tenants the obligations and costs of maintenance of the property. However, the *quid pro quo* is that in granting the lease, the tenants would be entitled to enjoy security of tenure throughout the term of the lease (and possibly beyond if it is granted within the 1954 Act). It will be recognised that it would be a huge mistake for the owners to expect their non-owning partners to contribute to the maintenance costs of the property (e.g. as expressed in the partnership agreement) without addressing the issue of occupation, as rights could automatically be implied, which may ultimately have a bearing on the value of the property and which would certainly be of significance in the event of a partnership dispute. Furthermore, in a worst case scenario, payment of substantial sums towards the maintenance of the building by non-owning GPs could potentially give them a claim to equitable ownership (*see* Example 1, p.69).

Occupation of surgery premises by third parties

It is essential to consider the position of each and every individual who crosses the threshold of the property to determine the basis upon which they enter and occupy. The position of the partners has been discussed above and the employees of the practice would not have any independent right to acquire security within the property as they fall under the wing of the partnership itself.

It can be presumed that patients enter the property as invitees (at least in the majority of cases!) and there would be no suggestion of any of them taking up long-term occupation. However, the position of others, ranging from pharmacists and dentists who may practice full time, to chiropodists and visiting consultants who may enter the property for one or two sessions per week, should be reviewed carefully in each case.

In *all* cases a legal form of document should be drawn up and signed *before* the first day of occupation. Failing this, the owners of the property are living on borrowed time as they may well find that if matters do not work out as they had hoped, claims may be brought against them. In such circumstances, quite apart from the immediate consequences of litigation and so on, this would do nothing to improve the relationship of the owner with his/her mortgagee who may seek to repossess the property in any event for breach of the terms of the mortgage. In nearly all cases, it will be necessary to seek the consent of the mortgagee before any third party takes up occupation of the property and this is certainly a point to check before the event rather than afterwards.

The need for a partnership agreement

It will already be apparent that a partnership agreement is necessary in order to declare the intention of the parties, for the benefit of each other in the first instance and, ultimately, as a declaration to the Court in the event of disputes which cannot be resolved amicably. However, there is a further reason why GPs should enter into a partnership agreement and that is to prevent a partnership at will (i.e. one without an agreement) being dissolved unilaterally and without notice. In the event of dissolution, the Partnership Act 1890 prescribes that *all* assets of the partnership shall be sold, and that includes the surgery premises, no matter which partners continue to occupy them and no matter whether there is negative equity or not. Accordingly, any partners who are contemplating surgery development should not be foolhardy enough to commit themselves to doing so before having first agreed their intentions with regard to the ownership/occupation of the property and, second, having ensured that those intentions are recorded in a properly drawn and legally enforceable agreement.

As the purpose of a partnership agreement is to create certainty in the minds of the partners, it can never be too detailed (no matter how many pages this may produce!). For example, if it is intended that not all the partners should be owners of the property, careful consideration should be given as to whether it is appropriate for any non-owning partners, who occupy under a mere licence, to pay for internal redecoration of the property. Whilst one partnership may consider it unfair on the owning partners for the non-owners to escape the cost of contributing to the cost of internal redecoration, in another partnership the owners may prefer to err on the side of caution and to absorb the cost of that responsibility themselves (lest in future years this may amount to evidence of the creation of a tenancy, notwithstanding the 'title' given to the arrangement).

It is essential that the agreement should deal with the following factors (described below) relating to the surgery premises:

- declaration of trust between the owners

- effect of retirement or death of an owning partner

- valuation of surgery premises

- consideration of mortgages

- rights of occupation of non-owning partners

- income/expenditure associated with the surgery premises

- consideration of the effect of the admission of a new partner in the future.

Declaration of trust

This is a declaration of the legal and equitable owners of the property and of their relevant shareholdings. It is particularly important where not all the partners have their names on the title deeds.

Effect of retirement or death of an owning partner

Upon the retirement or death of a partner it is most often the case that the outgoing partner will sell his/her share in the surgery premises to the remaining partners. This may take the form of a contractual obligation of sale (on the part of the outgoing partner) and purchase (on the part of the remaining partners) set down within the agreement or alternatively may be incorporated by way of cross options which have to be exercised within a specified period (e.g. 30 days after the date of retirement or death). The benefit of the latter scenario is that there are certain tax savings to be made in the event of death; however, the disadvantage is that the service of an option notice may be overlooked in the trauma of, for example, a partner's death, whereupon the only alternative may be that the partnership is dissolved after the prescribed period, which can lead to even greater uncertainty.

Without a declaration of intention within a partnership deed, the parties as joint owners have nothing to fall back on, other than the general legislation, which is not designed specifically to cater for the needs of GPs endeavouring to conduct their surgeries. Unless a dissolution of partnership is brought about, thus requiring the sale of all partnership assets (as discussed above), it may be difficult for an individual owner to secure the release of his/her capital. To do so, s/he may find him/herself being forced to issue proceedings under the Trust of Land and Appointment of Trustees Act 1996 which, having only recently been introduced, has not yet produced a body of case law to give guidance as to the likely interpretation of the Courts. Furthermore, in the case of a cost rented property, the forced sale of a property within a few years of development is most unlikely to produce a sum equal to the cost expended on it by the outgoing partner. Only compliance with a formula set down in a partnership agreement is likely to achieve this.

In the case of an outgoing partner who is faced with the prospect of crystallising a loss, s/he may prefer the alternative of remaining an owner of the property into the future, that is, as a non-partner, and to continue to enjoy the benefits of his/her share of the income from the property. Whilst the HA is not bound to pay rent to the outgoing partner, it would be the duty of the remaining partners, who are in receipt of the cost rent reimbursement, to pass to the outgoing partner his/her share, as s/he remains entitled to share in the income arising from his/her ownership of the property.

However, it cannot be pretended that this arrangement is ideal, for the following reasons:

- Once a partner has retired from the partnership, s/he can no longer claim business relief in respect of the property as a partnership asset as the property will be treated as an investment property. The ultimate disposal of the share therefore will not qualify for capital gains tax relief and it is possible that in future there may be a greater level of tax levied on the (unearned) income.

- Slowly, but surely, the position of the non-occupying owner will differ from those of the occupying partners. For example, if the roof is leaking, the temptation on the part of the non-occupying owner will be to have it patched. However, the occupying owner, who faces the prospect of water dripping on to his desk every day, may prefer a more substantial (and expensive) job to be undertaken.

In such circumstances, it is suggested that it would be essential for a formal lease to be drawn up, clarifying the position of both sides and dealing specifically with the responsibility (and costs) of maintenance.

Valuation of surgery premises

Valuation issues are almost worthy of a book in themselves. All that is certain at present is that there is no certainty as to the basis on which surgery premises should be valued. See pp. 85–91 for further details of the current position relating to valuation issues.

In the case of properties which are already owned by one or more of the partners, but which are to be 'substantially modified' by means of a cost rent extension, much of the value of the original building may be lost in the overall development. For example, a building originally worth £100 000 with conversion costs of another £100 000 may subsequently have an overall value of only £150 000.

If notional rent continues to be paid on the original part of the building and cost rent is paid in addition on the new building, the partners may wish to consider incorporating a 'phase I/phase II' basis of valuation into their partnership deed. This would have the effect of preserving the notionally rented value of the original building and taking into account separately the cost rented value added by the extension. However, this would not be viable where the HA wraps up the whole scheme into one new cost rent assessment as there would, in such circumstances, be no justification for isolating and preserving the value of the original building and the property would have to be treated as a whole for valuation purposes, with the principles of cost rent valuation applied as more particularly set down later (p.86).

Consideration should also be given to the effect of the use of grants or other 'free' monies which have been made available to the owners and the effect upon valuation.

Consideration of mortgages

Redemption of mortgages

Within your partnership agreement, in addition to dealing with the valuation issues as outlined above, you may wish to give specific consideration to the position relating to the treatment of the mortgage at the time of the transfer of a partner's share.

Whether you have a repayment or an endowment mortgage, if it is for a fixed rate of interest where a penalty would be payable in the event of early redemption (and assuming that you have locked into a similar rate of interest for the purposes of any cost rent reimbursement), you may prefer to specify that an incoming partner should be required to take over the share of the outgoing partner in the existing mortgage in order to avoid the prospect of the penalty becoming payable.

Cross-indemnities for mortgage liabilities

If each individual partner has his own personal mortgage arrangements in respect of his investment in the surgery (as was popular in order to secure tax advantages a few years ago), there may be a series of different charges registered against the title to the property. At the time of the original investment, and assuming equal shares of ownership, these are likely to have been for a similar sum and thus, to the extent the partners were cross-indemnifying each other, this was not unreasonable. However, upon a change in the partnership, in circumstances where the new partner wishes to offer his mortgagee the security of a legal charge against the title to the property, and in circumstances where the sum secured amounts to a greater sum than that of the other partners (as is inevitably the case as property values increase), the existing property owners should bear in mind that they are effectively indemnifying the new partner for his/her increased share of the borrowings. The reason for this is that even though an actual indemnity may not be entered into between the existing owners and the new mortgagee, in the event of the incoming partner failing to keep up his/her mortgage repayments, with the result that the mortgagees threaten to repossess, it is likely that the other partners would pay up the sum due rather than running the risk of the property being sold over their heads.

Treatment of endowment policies

In the case of endowment mortgages, it should be remembered that at the time of redemption, the amount of the original mortgage will not have reduced. However, in such circumstances it is relevant to consider the value of the endowment policy which provides collateral support to the mortgage.

In most cases, each borrower is likely to have his own endowment policy which is by far the simplest way forward. However, in a minority of cases, the original funding may have been set up on the basis of a policy effected on the lives of one or two of the partners only (as they were the cheapest to insure). In such circumstances, it is not only essential to include within the partnership agreement a declaration that such policies are for the benefit of *all* the owning partners in their respective shares (and the premiums associated therewith should be borne similarly) but it is also essential to provide for:

- an obligation on the part of the life-assured leaving the partnership to remain in contact, so that in the event of his/her death and at the time of maturity of the policy a claim may be made

- the basis of valuation of the policy in the event of one of the partners benefiting from the policy retiring from the partnership. This may be assessed on the simple value of the premiums paid or, the index-linked value, the LAUTRO value, the surrender value, or some other formula agreed, for example in discussion with the partnership accountants.

Term assurance policies

The same principle would apply with regard to any term assurance policies effected. It is not recommended to have term assurance on the lives of some partners and not others as this is one type of cover that all partners require equally. Once again, it should be borne in mind that if the premiums are payable by the partnership, then it will be the partnership that benefits from any proceeds paid out under the policy, and not the deceased partner's estate.

Rights of occupation of non-owning partners

The rights of occupation of partners who are not owners of the property should be dealt with by reference either to a separate lease or by the incorporation of a licence arrangement within the partnership agreement itself.

Income/expenditure associated with the surgery premises

It is most important to specify that all rent reimbursement received from the HA shall belong to the owning partners only and this should be reflected separately in the partnership accounts (*see* Example 2, on p.70). The distinction should also be clear between outgoings associated with the structure and fabric of the property (which should remain the responsibility of the owners) and day-to-day running expenses (which may be borne by the partnership as a whole).

Consideration of the effect of the admission of a new partner in the future

Whilst it is not possible to bind a future partner in the partnership within a present agreement (because a future partner would be required to sign the new agreement in order for it to be binding upon him/her), consideration may be given to the means of addressing this in the future.

A new partner being admitted to a practice would only be bound by a partnership agreement once it has been signed by all present partners. It is not sufficient simply to wave a copy of an out-of-date deed under the nose of an incoming partner and expect him or her to be bound by it by osmosis!

It is a common mistake to presume that a new partner is not truly a partner until the satisfactory completion of the probationary period. However, this can be an expensive mistake, as the new partnership commences on the first day of the incoming partner's probationary period. Accordingly, the agreement should be signed *prior* to that date.

It would be most unwise to permit the new partner to become a joint owner of the surgery premises before the satisfactory completion of the probationary period, as to do so would effectively thwart the other partners' ability to determine the partnership on grounds of unsuitability. However, it is not unknown for a new partner to agree to join the partnership on terms that s/he buys into a cost rent property at a level above open market value (whether it be based on any of the three methods of valuation discussed later, i.e. other than the Medical Practices Committee (MPC) basis) only to find that when the moment of truth arrives, s/he declines to do so, citing the basis of the MPC valuation as a justification. On the face of it, as the NHS Act creates a criminal offence, this could supersede the written word in a partnership agreement which provides civil remedies only, and in a worst case scenario, you could find yourselves stuck in a relationship with the new partner who insists contractually on purchasing a share of the property at only open market value. There are ways around this dilemma, however, and you should seek legal advice in order to overcome them.

Above all, it is essential to discuss and agree upon these issues in advance. Cases are known where partners have not been able to reach agreement on such issues and, accordingly, have rashly proceeded with a new surgery development whilst omitting all reference to such development from their partnership agreement! In other cases, partnerships which are on fairly rocky footings have elected to proceed with new schemes, suffering both the trauma and costs involved, in the expectation that this will serve to cement their partnerships. This is likely to be a pious hope and once the parties have been brought together under one new (and no doubt expensive) roof, it makes the problem of unravelling the partnership all the more difficult to resolve.

Valuation of surgery premises

Premises will require valuation where they have a capital value and, as has been seen, this can arise in the case of either a freehold or long leasehold. They may be funded either by notional rent or cost rent payable in accordance with paragraph 51 of the *Red Book*, and the valuation issues arising in each of these cases may be different.

Notionally rented surgery premises

It is an acknowledged principle that notional rent may, upon review, go down as well as up. Accordingly, in the case of a notionally rented property, there is no guaranteed income stream which may be relied upon at a given level in the future and as such it is presently considered by many to be inappropriate to base the open market valuation on the actual notional rent payable on the date of review.

In the case of notionally rented property, therefore, unless there is a lease in existence guaranteeing a level of rent to be assessed on an upwards-only basis for a term of years in the future, it is recommended that the property be valued in the open market with vacant possession.

GPs should then consider whether they wish the valuer to deem the use of the premises to be that of a GP surgery only (and if so whether this should be limited to NHS use) or whether the valuer may be instructed to take into account any alternative use which may be available subject to planning consent. Usually, it is considered fairer to limit the use to that of a NHS GP surgery as that is the basis upon which the DV assesses the notional rent for the purposes of authorising the level of HA reimbursement. However, in some cases, where there is a wider potential, owning GPs are anxious to retain the additional value which may be generated by taking such alternative use into account. The downside of this 'inflated value', however, is that it is unlikely to be possible to fund it solely from notional rent reimbursement, which could leave the partner who is due to purchase the share of an outgoing partner with a shortfall – perhaps not so attractive to an incoming partner.

Cost rented properties

The possibility of opening up the basis of valuation for a property constructed under the cost rent scheme is wider and a variety of arguments currently prevail, as set out below. These stem from a variety of interpretations of the NHS Act 1977 which provides, within section 54 and schedule 10, that it is a criminal offence for NHS GPs to buy and sell goodwill from each other.

Set out below is an example using assumed figures in order to demonstrate the application of the differing approaches.

Assume four partners develop new surgery premises in equal 25% shares as follows:

	Capital investment (total) [Capital (per partner)]	Income/Rent at assumed 10% (per partner)
Total actual cost	£1 000 000 [£250 000]	£100 000 [£25 000]
Approved HA cost	£800 000 [£200 000]	£80 000 [£20 000]
Open market value	£600 000 [£150 000]	£60 000 [£15 000]

The MPC view

The MPC takes a strict view of the NHS Act 1977 concerning sales of goodwill. It states that, without change to the existing statutory provisions, any transfer of partnership property between partners in an NHS general medical practice which involves a price or value in excess of the open market value with vacant possession is potentially open to challenge as involving a hidden sale of goodwill. Accordingly, in the given example, the MPC would not sanction any price in excess of £600 000.

This is the position they would adopt notwithstanding the fact the approved HA 'value' upon which the cost rent reimbursement was assessed is £800 000. Accordingly, this would force a retiring partner to crystallise his/her loss in the property and on a 25% share, s/he would have to find £100 000 capital in order to redeem his/her mortgage.

On the other hand, an incoming partner buying in at £150 000 would immediately become entitled to receive the retired partner's share of the cost rent at £20 000, which is likely to be more than is needed in order to service the loan.

In the writer's opinion, this does not present an equitable solution to the problem. Furthermore, it is suggested that if one considers the background against which the 1977 Act was introduced – it does not reflect the true interpretation of the Act. The legislation was introduced in order to prevent a retiring partner from seeking to include a goodwill payment within the sale price of ordinary surgery premises to his or her ongoing partners, knowing that they would need those premises in order to continue to see the patients of the practice. It will be appreciated that this situation is very far from the situation we are now considering, involving the sophisticated and complex nature of valuations undertaken with regard to surgery premises developed under the cost rent scheme.

The Hempsons view

At Hempsons we consider that even under the existing legislation (i.e. without amendment to the 1977 Act), it should be permissible for the property to be 'valued' based on the cost initially approved by the HA (i.e. £800 000 in the given example). In these circumstances, it has to be accepted that the outgoing partner would still crystallise a loss of £50 000 out of his/her original investment of £250 000 (although by retirement, s/he would hopefully either have reduced somewhat his/her share of the outstanding capital under a repayment mortgage, thus reducing the sum to be repaid at completion, or alternatively would have accumulated some capital in an endowment policy which may go some way towards redeeming the shortfall). The incoming partner should be in a position to raise the funds to buy the outgoing partner's share (based on his/her future entitlement to the cost rent reimbursement) on approximately a break-even basis, i.e. would borrow £200 000 against income of £20 000.

This appears to us to be a more equitable interpretation of the existing legislation.

It should be added that in certain cost rent schemes, where the partners have elected to construct a property which falls beyond cost rent limits, it may be possible to demarcate certain parts of the building as being 'private' for the purpose of a valuation. In these circumstances, there is no reason why the valuation of the 'private building' should not be added to the proposed 'cost rent valuation' basis described herein, thus increasing the overall value and reducing further (or completely) the loss to be borne by the outgoing partner.

Ideally, both the outgoing partner and the incoming partner should be put into a neutral position.

The RICS view

Recently the Royal Institution of Chartered Surveyors (RICS) introduced a revised basis of valuation for doctors' surgeries into its *Red Book* (not to be confused with the GP *Red Book*!). This is based upon the depreciated replacement cost of the building. The starting point is the sum it would cost to *replace* the building at the time of valuation (which, assuming there has not been a dramatic slump in the construction marketplace, is unlikely to be less than the original cost of construction). This figure is then *depreciated* to reflect those elements of the building which have a limited life expectancy (e.g. electrical wiring, pipework, etc.).

It will be seen that this valuation is based upon a mathematical calculation which has no bearing upon the open market value of the building. Whilst we at Hempsons recognise the validity of this basis of valuation, which is commonly recognised and used throughout the NHS marketplace (e.g. in the valuation of hospitals), we consider that it is more likely to be the subject of criticism pursuant to the NHS Act 1977 if ever it falls to be analysed by a Court in a test case, as it has no regard to either the open market value or the cost rent reimbursement.

'The GPFC view'

At a time when the GPFC was a government-owned body (i.e. before it was taken over by the Norwich Union), it was a requirement of its terms of lending to GPs undertaking cost rent schemes that such GPs entered into an agreement amongst themselves declaring that in the event of the retirement or death of a partner, his/her share should be valued at 'the higher of open market value or original cost'. It is readily apparent that this flies in the face of the MPC interpretation of the NHS Act 1977 and, accordingly, at one time, the views of two government bodies were directly contradictory!

Whilst we do not consider that the 'actual cost' argument stands up to scrutiny under the 1977 Act in cases where the cost of the building exceeded the original HA approved cost, we support the moral arguments behind it. This would allow, in our given example, a partner who had funded £250 000 of costs to be released from his/her obligations without suffering any shortfall. Indeed, if that partner's mortgage repayments had reduced the outstanding capital sum or if a capital fund had been built up in a policy, s/he might even be able to retire with a small amount of 'equity'. Accordingly, s/he would not be required to raise a capital sum to meet the shortfall payable to his/her mortgagee just at the time of retirement, when s/he wishes to consolidate his/her financial position for the future. Equally, the partner purchasing his/her share would be placed in exactly the same position as the other owning partners in the practice, namely that he would be funding a share costing £250 000 based on a cost rent reimbursement assessed at a 'value' of £200 000.

The justification behind this is that if the government (and indeed patients) expects GPs to provide improved accommodation and improved services, it is hardly reasonable to expect those very GPs who have sweated blood and tears and burned the midnight oil in order to get the scheme off the ground, to suffer a capital loss in the event of their retirement or death before the marketplace has allowed the value of the property to catch up with the cost. Furthermore, GPs' income often improves once the new surgery premises are available, thus allowing them to expand their range of services. This means that a new partner buying into the practice would benefit from the improved income from the outset and, unless he buys in at 'actual cost', he will not have participated in the full share of the capital required to produce that income.

As a matter of practice, we are aware of very many partnerships who have elected, and continue to elect, to incorporate this provision within their partnership agreement – and who would not have contemplated entering into the cost rent commitment in the first instance unless this provision had been agreed. On the basis that partners agree to be bound by the terms of the agreement without considering it necessary to refer the position to the MPC, there are many sales and purchases which have taken place, and which no doubt will continue to take place, without intervention from the MPC. Furthermore, to date there has not been one known prosecution arising under the NHS Act 1977.

The decision to switch from cost rent to notional rent

The cost rent income stream should (subject to one or two exceptions identified below) continue into the foreseeable future, that is until such time as the partners elect to convert to notional rent. Careful consideration should be given to the decision to convert from cost rent to notional rent because of the risk associated with a downward review of notional rent in the future. For this reason GPs should be careful to resist pressure applied by a HA to convert automatically to notional rent, which may at that moment appear more attractive and which gives the HA the benefit of reducing monies paid out of its cash-limited budget in the future. Once the switch has been made it is not possible to revert back to cost rent at a later date.

Preparation for the development phase

The golden rule is 'Planning Planning Planning' and you rush this at your peril! Attention to detail is essential whether you are dealing with negotiations with the vendor of a site, the agreement of a detailed specification with your architect, or agreeing the heads of terms with a third-party developer. If you do not allow yourselves adequate time it probably means that you are cutting corners, which may lead to problems in the future that are not always resolvable. Do not be rushed into signing anything as a result of pressure from anyone else, be it a commercial third party, your HA or even your solicitor(!), unless you are aware of and can afford to take the commercial risks. It is usually far better to allow yourself time to reflect on the scheme than to seek subsequently to dig yourselves out of a hole. On the other hand, there comes a point at which it is 'now or never' and you have to take the plunge; you shouldn't fear committing yourself at this point as long as you have built in adequate safeguards in the documentation and have considered their practical implications (i.e. whether they are likely to be worth the paper they are written on and whether, as a matter of practice, you would be able to afford to sue on the strength of them in order to protect your position).

You should seek relevant advice as early in the transaction as possible from your professional advisors when it is still possible for the scheme to be considered in the round and possibly restructured if it would be to your advantage to do so. This should not be perceived as 'making jobs for the boys', as a good professional advisor will be able to point you in the right direction and, more particularly, steer you away from any potential disasters. If you progress too much further along the path before seeking this advice, you may well find that you have incurred extensive costs before being made aware of the pitfalls and, possibly, that you feel you have committed to a certain course of action from which you cannot withdraw, notwithstanding the defects. Accordingly, as a preliminary to any further investigation, an early meeting should be arranged with the practice solicitor, the practice accountant and (subject to their go-ahead 'in principle') with your HA.

Having reached this stage you can then begin to search for a site (*see* Appendix B).

Early considerations

The site in question

Nearly every GP claims that there is a severe shortage of sites and that the one which is the subject of discussion is the only available site in the vicinity. Without wishing to appear cynical, this is by no means always the case and very often, where a site has to be dropped because problems become insurmountable, another preferable site is subsequently found. Don't be blinkered into thinking that the site presented to you is necessarily the only option, particularly if your gut reaction is to have some reservations about it.

If you are considering a new development, consider its proximity to your existing premises, taking into account the means of local transport available, the proposed availability of parking and other local competition. Patients can be surprisingly fickle when push comes to shove!

If you are considering developing an existing site, particularly under the cost rent scheme, consider the impact of the DV's valuation *at the time of acquisition of the site* upon the overall funding. Because this may pose an artificially low value, it may not only deny existing owning partners the opportunity to realise the equity they have already acquired in the site, but may produce insufficient funding for the scheme as a whole. In such circumstances it may be preferable to dispose of the original site and to invest elsewhere.

HA approval in principle

There is little point in pursuing the matter further without consultation with your HA to ensure, first, that it is willing to support your proposals for the identified site and, second, that it has the necessary funds available (*see* Chapter 1).

Disposal of existing site

If you are considering moving to a new site, consideration should also be given to the disposal of your existing site and to the funding of both sites simultaneously whilst the development phase is in progress. Negotiations with your HA at an early stage could give you added protection in this respect. Furthermore, a health service circular, which took effect from 1 April 1998, enables HAs to assist GPs who presently occupy leasehold property which is 'wholly inadequate' for modern general practice' to move to suitable alternative premises. This assistance could take the form of the payment of a reverse premium or dilapidation gain to enable the GPs to escape the lease.

The nature and viability of the scheme overall

Nobody in their right minds should willingly put themselves in a position where they are exposed to unnecessary or unreasonable development costs or find themselves trapped in an 'investment' without an escape route in the future. Your solicitor and accountant may be able to suggest an alternative structuring of the scheme which may prove to your advantage. For example, a GP who was intending to take on a lease without any capital value, and to develop a site at considerable cost to himself which would also have involved his personal exposure throughout the development phase (to costs in excess of £500 000), was very relieved when we produced an alternative scheme which not only had the effect of relieving him from the funding and development risks (by slotting in a third party to take such risks) but also offered him a lease on considerably less onerous terms for the future. In another case, where it was proposed that a group of GPs should purchase the freehold of a site which was situated over one of the main sewers leading into the city centre, it was agreed that a third party would purchase and develop the freehold of the site and sell it to the GPs at open market value at the conclusion of the scheme. This had the benefit not only of protecting the GPs from the development phase itself (coupled with the risk of fracturing the sewer!) but also of ensuring that they were not exposed to unrealistic costs which would not be covered, that would have left them with a negative equity for the future. In this particular case, this structure was made possible through the means of London Initiative Zone (LIZ) funding, which clearly would not apply outside London. However, if your legal and financial advisors are well versed in the NHS regulations, they may well be able to make proposals that are applicable to your particular area.

The short-term and long-term effects upon the partnership

There is no point in devoting extensive energy and resources into developing a scheme without considering the short- and long-term implications for your partnership. For example, if you are a single-handed practitioner who is developing a property under the cost rent scheme, you would be wise to seek assurances that the HA would be prepared to allow the cost rent to continue following your retirement from the practice. If there is a risk that your HA would cease cost rent funding in the event of your departure then you should seek to find another means of funding the scheme which will not put you in jeopardy at the time of your retirement. You cannot guarantee that because you have based your funding on an assumed 20-year term you will necessarily remain in the practice for that duration and it would be madness to allow yourself to face such problems (e.g. in the event of your forced early retirement on grounds of ill health).

Alternatively, if you are in partnership with a partner who is due to retire shortly, it may be advisable to proceed without including that partner within the scheme. This would entail ensuring that the other partners are capable of raising the additional share of funding themselves.

Considerations leading towards the development

From this point onwards a huge amount of your time will be required to make sure you get what you want. Do not be fooled into thinking this task can be delegated to a third party as, ultimately, only you can make the decisions with which you will have to live (and pay!) for the next 20 years or more. The matters you will need to consider at this stage are outlined below.

Agreement of heads of terms

Once you have taken preliminary advice from your professional advisors, and been given the go-ahead in principle, you can move to the next stage of seeking to negotiate heads of terms. These form the bones upon which the detailed 'flesh' may be added subsequently. At this stage you are likely to start to incur significant costs and one point you should consider is the prospect of whether any other parties will bear those costs for you.

If you have a surveyor negotiating heads of terms either with the vendor of a site or a third party who it is intended should purchase the site and develop it, your solicitor should seek to ensure that the terms remain conditional for as long as possible. If a conditional exchange of contracts can be effected so much the better, as this would give you the safeguard of knowing the site is secure whilst you have the opportunity to satisfy yourself on certain other criteria. As your 'satisfaction' is likely to incur you in further serious costs, it is just as well to know that the site will still be available at a predetermined price before you commit yourself to such expenditure. For example, you may seek to secure a conditional exchange of contracts subject to planning consent and a suitable offer of funding which itself would be linked to approval of a satisfactory tender.

Planning permission (outline)

An application for outline permission would relate principally to the change of use from whatever the present use of the site or building to a medical centre under class D(1)(a) of the Use Classes Order 1987. The detail of this has been dealt with in Chapter 2.

Funding offer (in principle)

Having received the go-ahead in principle from your HA, you will need to consider in greater detail the funding implications of the scheme you propose. At this stage, you will certainly not have available the detailed costing, but your valuer and architect should be able to give you some 'ball-park' figures within which to work to enable you to return to your practice accountant for more detailed advice and to make an approach to a lender.

Of course, it may be unnecessary for you to arrange the funding for yourselves as a scheme may be undertaken by a third-party developer who then agrees to grant a lease to you. In this case, it will be the developer who is funding the project and will be relying upon the payment of rent by your practice, throughout the term of the lease, to repay its borrowings. Essentially, if the developer can make a scheme viable based upon rent reimbursement available, there may be no good reason why you should not do so yourselves (although you may have to bear the VAT which a developer would be able to reclaim). However, there are many partnerships who consider that, because of the perceived problems of negative equity and the difficulties of encouraging incoming partners to buy a share, it is preferable to pursue a route of non-ownership through taking a lease. However, this approach may ignore the fact that a lease is not something that should be entered into lightly (as will be seen below), and it is recommended that the funding implications of undertaking the scheme personally should always be considered before this option is rejected.

If you are to pursue your own development, your HA may consider the alternative options of funding this through either the cost rent scheme or the notional rent scheme (possibly with the addition of an improvement grant). In recent years, the cost rent scheme has not been so popular as it proved to be increasingly inflexible, but with the recently published amendments, the funding produced by this scheme is likely to become more popular once again. However, the one big disadvantage of cost-rent developed surgeries will remain so long as there is uncertainty over the basis of valuations arising from it. For this reason, the option of pursuing a scheme which is funded through a combination of notional rent and an improvement grant may remain more popular, particularly as this entails you having to borrow (and thus repay) a smaller sum of money from the outset, thus reducing the risks involved.

Final considerations

1 Planning permission (detailed) and other approvals.

2 Negotiation of legal documentation.
   This will vary according to the nature of the scheme, as follows:
   (a) Ownership of the site
       (i) Option 1 – development of existing site.
           You may already own the site, in which case your solicitor will not need to investigate title on your own behalf. However, investigation of title will need to be undertaken on behalf of your mortgagee either by your own solicitor (if s/he is able to represent your mortgagee) or, more likely, by the mortgagee's independent legal advisors (in which case your solicitor will have to produce the evidence to satisfy them that your title is good and marketable).
       (ii) Option 2 – acquisition of a new site.
           Your solicitor will need to undertake a full investigation of title of the new site to ensure that there are no hidden defects which could restrict your development of it. The same investigation will need to be undertaken on behalf of your mortgagee, as discussed above.
           The principle of *caveat emptor* continues to apply under English law. This means 'let the buyer beware' and as such means that there is no obligation upon the vendor to disclose any defects relating to the property; it is for buyers to satisfy themselves that they are investing in something worthwhile. Problems may arise from a variety of different sources and as the answers are not immediately laid out in front of you, a 'problem' may

not disclose itself until your solicitor is some way down the track in investigating title.

Sometimes it may be possible to overcome problems; for example, in the case of a restrictive covenant seeking to restrict the use of the site and thus potentially thwarting your development plans, it may be possible to buy 'restrictive covenant indemnity insurance'. Your mortgagee will need to determine independently whether it will be satisfied by such a policy and this would, in any event, no doubt add to the costs of the development.

(b) Non-ownership/occupation.

If it is intended that you should not own the site but should occupy it under some other arrangement, normally a lease, it is likely that the proposed developer of the site, who will have to acquire the freehold (or superior leasehold) title itself, will wish you to enter into a commitment to take a lease of the site at the conclusion of the development phase. This will involve you entering into a document entitled an 'Agreement for Lease' or 'Development Agreement'.

In return for agreeing that you will guarantee to take a lease (which itself carries with it various onerous obligations – see below) you, in turn, will wish to ensure that the developer delivers what it has promised to deliver. This will entail annexing a detailed specification to the agreement, setting out, down to the last door handle, the detail of what you require. The terms you should seek in a development agreement are given in greater detail below.

3 Agreement of the Specification.

This has been touched on above, and whether or not you will own the building yourself, or are to take a lease, it is essential that you should pay enormous attention to the detail of the specification. Whilst a cheaper construction may appear initially to your advantage, you should consider also the longer-term implications with regard to maintenance. As a generalisation, cheaper products are likely to require greater maintenance and earlier replacements in the future and you should remember that all such costs are likely to come out of your own pocket rather than being funded through either cost rent or notional rent/improvement grant from the outset. They are also likely to lead to a lower valuation of the property overall. Certainly the quality and standard of the fixtures and fittings are something which the DV is likely to take into account when assessing the rental value of such a property.

It is worth your while undertaking a certain amount of research of the products to be used (e.g. by talking to other GPs who have already been through the exercise themselves). This is your opportunity to learn from others' mistakes!

4   Building contract.

If you are undertaking the development yourself, you will need to enter into a contract with the building contractor. This will take the form of either a JCT Contract or a design and build contract.

Under a JCT Contract, you will be able to retain greater control over the ultimate design of the building but will not have an absolute guarantee with regard to the costs. Whilst the contractor will agree to undertake the development at a pre-determined figure, that figure may be adjusted further as a result of other contingencies which arise throughout the development phase.

A design and build contract gives you absolute certainty as to the cost. However, in entering into such a contract, effectively you are delegating the design element of the building to the contractor, who will doubtless be looking for ways to cut corners in order to save money. In one such scheme, for example, the contractor elected to save money on the provision of steel girders by using a reduced number of larger girders with the result that the ceiling height was 18 inches lower than the GPs had expected.

You should seek advice from your architect as to the best way forward in each case.

5   Collateral warranties.

In order to safeguard your position *vis-à-vis* third parties who will be contributing to the construction of your property, you need to ensure that you have a direct contractual link with them. Unless there is something declared in writing, you cannot assume that this link exists (and even if it does exist, and you can establish that a duty of care is owed to you, it is generally far more difficult to establish a claim in negligence than for a breach of contract).

To this end, you should ensure that you have collateral warranties (contracts) with each of the relevant design sub-consultants and professionals who are working on your scheme. Your architect should be able to produce a list of all such parties and your solicitor can advice on the form of warranties you should enter into.

It is essential to ensure that all relevant parties have adequate indemnity insurance so that in the event of you being forced to sue them, you will not find you have an empty claim on the basis you are suing 'a man of straw'. Claims arising in respect of defects in the construction or design of the property are likely to be substantial and if you are unsuccessful in extracting money from the relevant party, you will have to bear such costs yourselves.

6   HA commitment to the project.
Finally, once all other steps have been undertaken, you should return to your starting point and secure final approval from the HA. At this point, you should put your position in writing and make it absolutely clear that you are only prepared to commit yourself to the project in hand based on the HA backing and the assurance that you will continue to receive cost rent/notional rent at a level not less than the figure upon which you have been basing your calculations.

There are recent examples of cases where HAs have produced an interim cost rent statement to GPs and have started off by paying that figure in the form of cost rent reimbursement, but subsequently have sought to renege on it (usually as a result of later investigation by their auditors). This has occurred, for example, in cases where HAs have agreed historically that it would be wise to 'plan for the future' by allowing for an additional consulting room. Subsequently, the auditors have criticised this policy and sought to reclaim the 'overpayment' of cost rent reimbursement. Hopefully, the implementation of the new Cost Rent Regulations which encourage 'planning for the future' will prevent this from being repeated in the future. However, in such cases, had there been written evidence in the form proposed above, the HA would have found itself in greater difficulty in seeking to reclaim earlier 'overpayments' based on the evidence of the intention of the parties at the time.

Consideration of Development Agreement and Lease

We have discussed arrangements for the development of properties which involve third parties. These may or may not come under the heading of 'private finance initiatives' (PFI). Many of those which do involve private finance are not officially classified as PFIs and indeed, the only finance involved is that borrowed by the developer which is to be wholly repaid through means of rent reimbursement payable via a lease (i.e. the developer has not contributed any of its own private capital at all).

A developer will usually require a lease of 20–25 years to be entered into by GPs, as it is over this term of years that its funding is arranged. Accordingly, the developer is likely to seek to ensure that a GP practice remains in occupation of the new surgery throughout that term of years, thus ensuring a steady income stream which is effectively government backed (i.e. rent reimbursement paid by the HA to the GPs who are under a contractual obligation to pay it to the developer/landlord). When considering entering into such a scheme, therefore, you should be well aware of the fact that the surgery has to be built to last and should, hopefully, be sufficiently flexible to allow for variations in the future (although these are unlikely to be guaranteed from the outset).

It is essential to remember that, whilst you may work closely with the developer in working up a scheme over a period of months or even years, the personalities involved are 'not on your side' and, for this reason, it is essential that you should take independent advice to ascertain the true strength of your position.

Set out below is a list of some of the more essential points which should be found in any Development Agreement and subsequent Lease. However, this should not be regarded as an exhaustive list and it is essential that careful consideration should be given to the circumstances of each case.

Development Agreement

1 Requirement for developer to seek detailed planning consent at its own cost in accordance with plans agreed with the GPs; to supply GPs with copies of the application and supporting plans, and to keep them up to date with progress reports.

2 Requirement for the developer to appeal against the rejection of such application or the imposition of any unreasonable conditions.

3 Requirement for the developer to apply for and comply with any other necessary consents such as:

- listed building approval

- building regulation approval

- fire officer's approval

- health and safety compliance

- any superior landlord's approval.

4 Agreement of form of detailed specification (to be annexed to the Development Agreement).

5 Agreement of form of building contract and deeds of collateral warranty with design sub-consultants to be annexed to the Development Agreement.

6 Requirement for the developer to ensure that the building contractor carries out the development:

- in a good and workmanlike manner diligently and expeditiously
- in accordance with detailed planning permission
- in accordance with requisite consents
- in accordance with all relevant codes of practice or British Standards
- in accordance with the building contract
- in accordance with the specification.

7 Requirement for the building contractor to maintain adequate insurances and to note the interests of all relevant parties.

8 Ability for the GPs to appoint an independent monitoring surveyor who should be entitled to inspect the works and to attend project meetings and in particular who should have the right to make written representations and require the removal of works which don't comply with the obligations entered into.

9 Right for the monitoring surveyor to be able to issue a list of works required to be undertaken before the written statement of practical completion is finally issued.

10 Right for the monitoring surveyor to agree to a list of defects to be rectified within the defects period (e.g. 12 months).

11 Copy of the written statement of practical completion to be given to the GPs.

12 Copy of the final form of plans and specifications together with working manuals and documents to be provided to the GPs.

13 Access to the GPs to undertake fitting-out works before final completion of the Lease, i.e. before the rent becomes payable.

14 Grant of lease to take place within a specified number of days following the issue of the certificate of practical completion and GPs to take up occupation.

15 Provision for the termination of the agreement in the event of failure on the part of the developer to comply as above.

16 Arbitration.

Lease

A lease takes the form of a contract between the landlord and the tenant. You should be aware that the identity of the landlord may change at any time and without prior notice to you. You should not rely therefore upon the personality of the prospective landlord with whom you have been negotiating when considering the implications of the application of the terms of the lease.

A lease normally follows a reasonably set pattern (although not a set form) but you should ensure that the following are included:

1 Description of the premises. In the case of premises which form part of a larger structure, or in a case where the landlord is accepting responsibility for maintenance of certain parts of the premises, the extent of the premises should be defined clearly with regard to:

- identifying the parts which belong to you

- identifying those parts for which you are responsible for ongoing maintenance

- identifying those parts of the building for which the landlord is to be responsible.

2 Rights associated with the demise, to include:

- rights of way

- rights to use car parking spaces

- rights to the free passage of services (drainage, water, gas, electricity, etc.)

- rights to erect signs outside the premises

- rights to have access to other property for the purposes of maintenance

- right of access by ambulances

- rights for the disposal of refuse (and clinical waste).

3 Rights over your property exercisable by third parties, for example the right of the landlord to enter your property for the purposes of maintaining other parts of the building or for the purposes of inspection. You should endeavour to ensure that such rights are exercised only outside usual surgery hours by prior appointment.

4 Tenant's covenants (i.e. obligations imposed upon you). You should check carefully the following:

- Alienation (i.e. rights for you to dispose of your interest in the property). You should seek to ensure that an individual tenant has the right to assign the lease to another GP-tenant without the need for the landlord's consent or any ongoing obligations following his/her retirement.

- User. Naturally you will require the right to use the property for the purposes of a medical centre. For your own purposes, it would be wise to ensure as wide a use as possible to give you flexibility. However, you should be aware this can have adverse repercussions in the context of subsequent rent reviews. It would probably be unwise to accept any restriction upon the use of the premises for NHS purposes only as nobody can envisage how the NHS system in this country will operate in the future. Any necessity for you to obtain consent to change the use under the lease in the future could necessitate you having to pay a premium to your landlord at the time in order to enable you to obtain such consent.

- Liability for maintenance. Ideally you should endeavour to negotiate liability for internal non-structural redecoration only. This would leave the landlord with the maintenance of the structure and exterior at its own expense, i.e. without charging a service charge. Alternatively, if you are required to take on full repairing and insuring (FRI) liability, you should ask your surveyor to negotiate a supplemental payment of rent reimbursement pursuant to paragraph 51, schedule 4, paragraph 2 (ii)(g) of the *Red Book*. This would be relevant either in circumstances of you having to undertake this responsibility yourselves or where you have to contribute to the cost through a service charge.

5 Insurance. The Landlord will doubtless wish to insure the property, albeit at your expense. The cost of this should form part of your rent reimbursement as permitted under paragraph 51 of the *Red Book*. In the event of the premises being damaged (in circumstances where you are not responsible and thus liable to pay for the cost of reinstatement yourselves), the lease should state that the rent will abate until such time as the landlord has used the monies received from the insurance company to reinstate the premises. Furthermore, it would be wise to seek the right for you to terminate the lease in the event of the premises not having been reinstated within a specified period (e.g. 12 months). Failing this, you would be unable to enter into the commitment of taking on secure alternative permanent accommodation for yourselves elsewhere.

6 Rent review. Ideally, there should not be an 'upwards only' provision within the lease and the rent payable should be tied in exactly to that approved by the DV. However, even in cases where landlords are prepared to accept this proposal, it is unusual for them to be prepared to allow the rent to go down to a level below that agreed initially, at the time of the grant of the lease, as that figure would usually represent the minimum sum required in order to guarantee the repayment of their funding.

   In circumstances where a landlord (or its mortgagee) is not prepared to accept such a proposal, you should seek to avoid the possibility of you being exposed to a downwards review by the DV at a time when the landlord seeks to review the rent upwards by a small amount. There are ways around this which you should discuss with your legal adviser.

In summary, a lease without any capital value (i.e. one where current market rental is paid to the landlord each year) should always be regarded foremost as a liability. Whilst negotiations may lead to the terms of a specific lease being as 'user friendly' as possible, ultimately the fact remains that the tenant will be liable not only to pay rent throughout the term but, in addition, to return the building to the landlord in tip-top condition at the end of the term at his/her own expense. Furthermore, it will not be possible for the tenant to break the contract early before the end of the term without the landlord's approval. Accordingly, whilst there may be very strong reasons for partners to enter into a lease with, for example, a property developer, it should not necessarily be regarded as the soft option. Furthermore, it is very often the case that if the property developer can make a profit out of the development, it is possible for you to do so also. Conversely, if the figures do not stack up for you, it is unlikely you will find a developer who is prepared to take over the project on your behalf.

The future

The impact of primary care groups (PCGs) upon medical centre developments is as yet an unknown and untested field. Assurances are presently being given by the NHS Executive that the payment of rent and rates will continue unhindered. However, it is already clear that decisions concerning issues such as improvement grants will be subject to board approval and it will be interesting to see how the members of the board elect to cast their votes. It remains to be seen whether a board member can be sufficiently objective to vote in favour of a decision which will positively benefit a rival practice to his own down the road.

It seems likely that the impact of PCGs will lead to the creation of larger practice units with the knock-on implications for the surgery premises housing those units. It can only be imagined that the need for the sort of advice contained within this book will become ever greater!

This chapter has been written in accordance with the laws of England and Wales as at the date of publication.

4

The financial viewpoint

SEAMUS KEHOE

In the initial stages when GPs are investigating the possibilities of embarking on a new cost or notional rent development, they should bear in mind that while it is possible to arrange most loans where the interest in its entirety is covered by the cost or notional rent, the GPs will personally have to make provisions for the capital repayment from their own resources. Agreement should also be reached on the apportionment of any abortive costs, should the development not proceed to fruition for any reason. These costs can be substantial, depending at what stage of the proceedings the development falls through. It is therefore imperative that the practice is aware of exactly what cost will be incurred in respect of legal and architectural fees, and so on, at the different stages of the development. It has been known for partnerships to split acrimoniously over who is responsible for such costs. Litigation is costly and can be a long drawn out procedure which seldom has any winners. Having a legally binding agreement in place could prevent such problems from happening in your practice.

Costs to be budgeted for

- **Survey fees:** where a greenfield site is involved, many lenders will not require a valuation; others are prepared to pay for their own survey. In these circumstances, as long as the team involved with the project has sufficient professional indemnity, you will normally have adequate protection should the workmanship prove to be faulty. Where a building is being purchased for modification, a survey should always be undertaken to assess the condition of the existing building and its foundations.

- **Legal fees:** you will be responsible for your own solicitor's costs, and in most instances, for those of the lender in connection with both the mortgage and the conveyance of the property.

- **Arrangements and commitment fees:** most lending sources will make a charge for arranging a loan and some will make a charge on any amount of the loan that is not taken up within a certain timescale. Such fees are normally negotiable.

- **Cost of surrendering existing lease or sale of existing property:** most lenders will be prepared to roll these costs into the new scheme.

- **Removal costs**

- **Furniture and equipment:** furnishing and equipping a new surgery will be a direct expense on the practice. Tax relief can be claimed by way of capital allowances on fixtures and fittings. It is important therefore to identify any furnishings which are classed as fixtures and included in the building, in order that the relevant capital allowances can be claimed on them. At some future date these items will need replacing. To minimise the effect on the partnership and new partners in particular, serious consideration should be given to setting up a 'sinking fund' to replace or upgrade such expensive items as computers, and so on. All users, whether property owners or not, should contribute to the fund in proportion to their use of the premises.

  Most lending sources will be prepared to lend up to 15% of building costs for furniture and equipment at their standard rates. Care should be taken when considering the loan term for such additional amounts, as you will not want to have to service an outstanding debt after the items concerned have passed their 'sell-by date'. Normally such loans should be set up on a variable rate basis for ease of early repayment should the practice wish to do so at some future date.

- **Negative equity:** should there be a negative equity situation with the existing building, most lending sources will be prepared to consider rolling all or part of the amount involved into the new loan arrangement.
- **Fire insurance on the building and contents:** this should include cover for the loss of cost/notional rent during the rebuilding period. The master policies offered by some lenders can provide good value for the premium charged.
- **Engineer's report:** a soil survey report should be carried out before exchange of contracts to ensure that there is no contamination. This should also show up any hidden subterranean problems that would make it more expensive to erect a building on the site. Any existing building on the site, even if it is to be demolished, should be examined for the presence of deleterious materials within the structure. The presence of such substances as asbestos in large quantities would make demolition a very costly exercise. The cost of sorting out any problems, including soil contamination, that are highlighted in such reports should be reflected in a reduced purchase price.
- **Architect and quantity surveyor's costs:** the bulk of professional costs will be on the architectural side, but as there is a lot of competition for GP surgery business, it is possible to have some of the initial work carried out by an architect for a minimal fee. This is on the understanding that should you decide to proceed with the project, you will appoint that person to the project. Some architectural firms will have their own in-house quantity surveyor, which can make the overall package on offer very competitive. The cost for architect's services, depending on the size of the project, will be negotiable. When appointing an architect, make sure that the people you intend to use have experience in developing GP surgeries. Speak to other GPs who have been involved in similar proceedings and find out how their working relationship developed with the various professionals they appointed to their team. Changing architects during the project can be a very costly exercise.

- If you are effecting a new loan with an existing lender it should be possible to negotiate an improvement on any existing interest rates that are out of line with the market at that time.

Once you have decided to embark on the scheme, you should then give consideration to finding a suitable lending source. The main players in the surgery financing market have regional consultants who offer specialist advice on surgery projects.

The advice offered will normally be of a high standard, but can vary from company to company and region to region depending on the experience of the individual. It is, however, worth remembering that they will inevitably only give you advice based on their own company's terms as it is their products that they are employed to sell. This could result in a conflict of interest when a doctor is looking for the cheapest possible interest rate and the provider is looking to maximise profitability.

The specialist independent financial advisor (IFA) on the other hand can review the total market and offer the doctors the best choice of loan available at any one time without having any vested interest in that choice. Most loans take many months from the initial application to the completion of the deal, and it is a fact that the company offering the most competitive package when you first submit your application may not necessarily be the one offering the best terms when you come to complete the loan. An IFA will continue to monitor the market and keep you appraised of changing terms and interest rates, thus ensuring that the loan that you eventually complete on is the most competitive package available at that time.

The IFA can advise you on the complete package, including the repayment vehicle that is best suited to your personal requirements. If you are dealing directly with the lending source, the advice regarding the loan repayment will normally be given via a referral to their direct sales force, who may not be so well versed with GP requirements in relation to surgery projects.

In either case, you will not normally be charged a fee, since the consultant will receive the remuneration directly from the company as either a basic salary or a combination of basic salary and commission over-ride. The IFA receives his/her remuneration from an insurance company based on insurance or investment products that may be sold in connection with the loan. Ultimately, the person you choose to deal with should be one that you personally feel comfortable with (be they a particular lender's consultant or a specialist IFA) and one that can advise you on all aspects of the cost/notional rent schemes and the availability of products that can meet your requirements. After all, it is not always possible for doctors to be aware of the financial intricacies involved. It should be the function of the financial advisor to furnish you with as much relevant information as is available, and to assist you in making an informed decision.

Repayment methods

There are three main types of mortgage available in the market place, namely: capital and interest repayment mortgage; interest only mortgage; and evergreen mortgage. These are described below.

- *Capital and interest repayment mortgage:* under this method, the monthly payment to the lender will pay off both the loan (the capital) and the interest on the loan.

- *Interest only mortgage:* this is a repayment method whereby only the interest on the loan is paid to the lender each month, whilst making a separate payment into an investment vehicle to pay off the capital at the end of the term. The investment vehicle is normally an endowment policy, pension, or personal equity plan (PEP), or individual savings account (ISA). Some lending institutions will also accept a portion of the loan being paid from the NHS superannuation (NHSS) tax-free cash.

- *Evergreen mortgage:* with an evergreen loan the lender does not require the loan to be repaid by any specific date, so the only cost to the borrower is the monthly interest.

The repayment method best suited to an individual's needs will depend on each person's personal and financial circumstances. Some of the main considerations that should be taken into account in reaching that decision follow.

Both cost and notional rent are treated as earned income within the practice and as such attract basic and higher rate tax. Unlike residential mortgages, a business loan attracts tax relief on the total interest paid each year at the highest marginal rates paid by the partners. As a rough rule of thumb, in any one fiscal year the partners will pay tax on the difference between the cost/notional rent received and the interest paid on the surgery loan. Conversely, they will receive tax relief on any interest payments over and above the cost/notional rent.

A capital and interest repayment mortgage has the benefit of guaranteeing that your mortgage will be paid off at the end of the term. The main disadvantage is that it does not maximise tax relief on the loan interest. The gross amount of each instalment remains the same through the term of the loan but the balance of capital and interest changes from year to year as the loan amount reduces. Tax relief is only available on the interest content of each instalment, therefore, the net amount payable increases each year over the term of the loan.

The figures given in Table 4.1 illustrate the split of capital and interest on a £100 000 loan over 25 years at an 8% fixed interest rate and a cost rent reimbursement rate of 8%, assuming that the project is fully cost rented. Over the 25-year term, the total amount of tax paid on the loan of £100 000, after taking into account the cost rent at 8% and a marginal tax rate of 40%, would be £27 189. Due to the fact that most of the tax relief has been used up in the early years of a repayment loan, it may be difficult to persuade a new incoming partner to take over such a loan which, because of the tax position, will be an increasing drain on their cash flow. This could result in the outgoing partner having to redeem their portion of the existing loan, thereby incurring possible redemption penalties.

In the example shown, if the loan is continued to maturity, the practice, under current tax regulations, will have paid on average £1087 in extra taxes each year. Should higher rate tax margins increase in the future, this figure would become even greater. If we assume that in year 10 the marginal tax rate has been increased to 60% for the balance of the term, then the tax payable in year 10 would increase from £564.85 to £846.97, and in year 20 from £1865.80 to £2798.70. Conversely, if the marginal

Table 4.1: Capital and interest repayment schedule

Year	Annual repayment	Capital repaid	Capital outstanding	Interest repaid	Tax paid[a] at 40%
1	9 281.08	1 320.03	98 679.97	7 961.05	15.58
2	9 281.08	1 428.84	97 251.13	7 852.24	59.10
3	9 281.08	1 546.63	95 704.50	7 734.45	106.22
4	9 281.08	1 674.11	94 030.39	7 606.97	157.21
5	9 281.08	1 812.11	92 218.28	7 468.97	212.41
6	9 281.08	1 961.48	90 256.80	7 319.60	272.16
7	9 281.08	2 123.18	88 133.62	7 157.90	336.84
8	9 281.08	2 298.20	85 835.42	6 982.88	406.85
9	9 281.08	2 487.64	83 347.78	6 793.44	482.62
10	9 281.08	2 692.70	80 655.08	6 588.38	564.65
11	9 281.08	2 914.67	77 740.41	6 366.41	653.44
12	9 281.08	3 154.93	74 585.48	6 126.15	749.54
13	9 281.08	3 414.99	71 170.49	5 866.09	853.56
14	9 281.08	3 696.51	67 473.98	5 584.57	966.17
15	9 281.08	4 001.22	63 472.76	5 279.86	1 088.06
16	9 281.08	4 331.04	59 141.72	4 950.04	1 219.98
17	9 281.08	4 688.07	54 453.65	4 593.01	1 362.80
18	9 281.08	5 074.52	49 379.13	4 206.56	1 517.38
19	9 281.08	5 492.82	43 886.31	3 788.26	1 684.70
20	9 281.08	5 945.59	37 940.72	3 335.49	1 865.80
21	9 281.08	6 435.71	31 505.01	2 845.37	2 061.85
22	9 281.08	6 966.21	24 538.80	2 314.87	2 274.05
23	9 281.08	7 540.45	16 998.35	1 740.63	2 503.75
24	9 281.08	8 162.03	8 836.32	1 119.05	2 752.38
25	9 281.08	8 836.32	0.00	444.76	3 022.10

[a]This is tax paid at 40% on the difference between cost rent and interest repayments.

rate drops below 40% in the latter years, the tax bill would be reduced.

A capital and interest repayment mortgage does not automatically provide life insurance. To ensure that the loan is paid off on death, the borrower will need to effect at least a mortgage protection policy. Consideration should also be given to critical illness cover which would pay off the mortgage should the borrower suffer from any of a number of illnesses, such as cancer, heart attack or multiple sclerosis, to name but a few. If you are considering such a contract, the definition of insured perils is of the utmost importance. To ensure that you are made aware of the full range of contracts that are available, you should contact an IFA, who will assess the whole marketplace on your behalf.

The structure of a repayment mortgage is such that it is not until half way through the mortgage term that the borrower starts to make real inroads into the actual amount of the capital that is repaid, as can be seen in the 'capital outstanding' column of Table 4.1. Therefore, if one of the partners were to leave the practice after a period of – say – 10 years, they may be surprised at the small proportion of the actual loan that has been paid off. Another point worth remembering is that unless there is capital appreciation in the building, the only money the outgoing partners will receive from the incoming partner will be a return of the capital that has been repaid over the years, with no allowance for inflation or interest. As the money will not have the same purchasing power then, in real terms, the outgoing partner will, in fact, have suffered a loss on the investment. That said, one should not just view a new surgery project merely on a financial level. An up-to-date work environment will reduce the stress and strain of day-to-day surgery work, thereby improving the partners' overall quality of life.

With an interest only mortgage, the borrower will pay the interest to the lender each year, and under current legislation will receive tax relief on this figure at the highest marginal rate payable by the practice. This will maximise the tax relief over the term of the loan. As long as the interest paid matches the cost/notional rent payable, there will be no tax liability. As the tax relief is spread evenly over the term of the loan, most new incoming partners would feel happier taking over an 'interest only' loan which would continue to enjoy maximum tax relief throughout its term rather than the decreasing tax relief available under a repayment loan. Assuming the new partner takes over the existing loan on identical interest rate terms, this would avoid the worry of the outgoing partner having to pay a redemption penalty. The capital can be repaid by any combination of endowment, PEPs, ISAs or the tax-free cash from a personal pension or the NHSS. With all of these methods the borrower would need to ensure that the assumed growth rate is a realistic one and not merely the highest rate that the company can legally quote. When assessing the companies to use for these products, the borrower should look at the financial strength of the recommended company as well as its past performance record and charging structure. Some lending sources will insist that you use their insurance products. These may not be as competitive as others on the market. This fact should be taken into consideration when assessing the overall competitiveness of the loan.

Past performances are no guarantee of future payments and if the assumed growth rate is not achieved, the borrowers will have to find the shortfall from their own resources. Should the chosen investment outperform the assumed growth rate, then any remaining surplus, after redeeming the mortgage, will be returned to the borrower. This will normally be free of personal taxation. The monthly payments relating to the investment vehicle chosen to repay the loan will remain constant throughout the term and should the borrower move from one surgery to another, the policy can be transferred to the new loan. This would ensure that at least part of the new loan would be paid off when the original policy matures. Any balance would need to be covered by a new policy which would normally be taken out to retirement age.

The most popular means of repaying an interest only loan is a minimum cost endowment policy. This automatically provides life cover, with the investment return providing the cash sum to pay off the loan at maturity. The new style unit-liked endowment contract provides a wide range of investment funds from low to high risk and has some very attractive add-on options, which can provide extra cover such as critical illness at a much keener rate than if the critical illness contract was taken out on a stand-alone basis.

From April 1999, PEPs will no longer be available for new investment money. Current PEP investments will, however, be allowed to exist as separate tax-efficient investments outside the chancellor's new individual savings account (ISA) which will replace them. When ISAs replace PEPs and tax-exempt special savings accounts (TESSAs), savers will be allowed to invest a maximum of £7000 in ISAs in the first year, followed by £5000 per year over an initial guaranteed period of 10 years. On the known facts, ISAs would appear to be a suitable repayment alternative to PEPs. When the new rules on ISAs are finalised, existing PEP borrowers should assess their position and take whatever corrective measures are required to make sure that their mortgage will be repaid at the end of the term. Personal pension policies, which currently attract both tax relief on premiums at the highest marginal rate paid and enjoy considerable tax savings on their investment funds, are the most tax efficient means of repaying a mortgage.

At maturity, in addition to the tax-free cash that is used to pay off the loan, there will normally be a substantial pension payable to the borrower for life. Because the borrower is funding for both tax-free cash and pension, at first glance this method of repaying a loan can seem expensive. However, when the premiums are netted down after tax relief and compared pound for pound with the return made on other forms of investment, it will be realised that personal pension plans (PPPs) have no equal as an investment opportunity. If a GP is planning to retire early, s/he should give serious consideration to the use of a personal pension plan to repay the surgery loan.

Although GPs receive the majority of their income from the NHS, they are taxed under schedule D on that income. They are thus in the unique position of having the option of pensioning their NHS earnings twice. Most GPs are members of the NHSS scheme. They pay 6% of their 'superannuable' earnings to the NHSS scheme. In addition, subject to Department of Social Security (DSS) agreement, they may elect to pay up to 9% by way of additional voluntary contributions (AVC) in order to secure 'added years' service and/or additional pension by means of AVC or free-standing AVC (FSAVC) policies. Tax relief is granted on these contributions on a concessionary basis known as the A9 concession. If a GP wishes to forego the concessional tax relief on his/her total contribution to the NHSS scheme, this does not affect the benefit they receive under the scheme. It does, however, allow them to pay contributions into a PPP based on their net relevant earnings from all sources. This allows the GP to pension the same earning twice whilst only claiming tax relief on the PPP contributions. The amount payable under the PPP would be subject to normal Inland Revenue maximums.

The decision to forego tax relief can be changed from year to year to suit personal circumstances. Should this option be decided on, the GP should notify – in writing – both the health authority (HA) and the Inland Revenue tax inspector concerned.

Alternatively, if a GP has earnings over and above the NHS superannuable income, he or she may effect a PPP for the balance of that income.

The amount of money available is calculated by subtracting the superannuable income in any one tax year from his or her net relevant earnings in that same tax year. Net relevant earnings (NRE) will consist of earned income from all sources less expenses allowed under schedule D. The NRE can be increased for pension purposes for group practices by setting the surgery loan up on a personal basis and claiming the tax relief on the loan interest via the GP's personal tax return. The main drawback of a personal loan is that tax relief will cease immediately the GP leaves the practice. Therefore in a practice where loans are set up on an individual basis, or a combination of individual loans and partnership loans, the procedure to be followed on a partner's departure from the practice will need to be dealt with separately under the partnership deed for each loan type. Where the loan is being taken over by the practice or the new incoming partner, care needs to be taken that the lending source does not treat it merely as a book entry, which could have serious tax implications for the existing partnership or the new partners.

The NRE would normally be subject to the earnings cap which is one of the limiting factors when assessing the maximum pension contribution payable in any one year. Should the PPP route be chosen, it is imperative that expert advice is sought from someone who understands all the options available and their implications for the GP's within their overall personal financial strategies.

An evergreen loan maximises the tax relief on the loan interest in the same way that an interest only loan does. The attraction of this particular type of loan is that there is no need to make provision for the repayment of the capital.

This allows the borrower extra cash to plan his or her investment and retirement strategy without having regard to the extra restrictions imposed by tying it in with the surgery mortgage. When the time comes for the GP to leave the surgery, for whatever reason, the new incoming partner simply takes over the outgoing partner's share of the existing loan and raises a further loan for any additional equity that may have accrued in the building.

'Capital holidays' are another useful vehicle for consideration. These can be agreed with some lending sources for any period from one to 15 years. During the capital holiday period the practice pays the interest only to the lending source, with no provision being made for the capital repayment of the proportion of the loan that is on the capital holiday. An example of where this might be used to keep partners' cost down would be where the senior partner is within a few years of retirement and does not wish to get involved in the scheme, where a practice is expected to expand the number of partners over the coming years, or where there is a substantial part of the loan interest which is not covered by the cost of notional rent payment. In the first two instances, the amount of the loan put on a capital holiday would equate with the share of the loan that would be taken over by the incoming partner and the latter would be the amount of the loan not serviced by the cost or notional rent income. The capital holiday in addition to keeping each partner's cost to a minimum, would also maximise tax relief on the loan interest during the capital holiday period on the portion of the loan that was on the capital holiday.

Capital holidays and evergreen loans are not always on offer from all lending sources and may have to be specially negotiated to fit each practice's circumstances. The lender may also impose some special conditions on such loans.

Fixed or variable rate loan?

Depending on whether you are seeking cost or notional rent reimbursement, there will be a number of considerations before deciding on which path to follow.

Cost rent

If money for the surgery project is borrowed on a variable rate basis, then the cost rent will be reimbursed on a variable basis.

Should the money be raised from the practice's own resources or be borrowed on a fixed rate basis, then the reimbursement will be on a fixed basis. The decision to follow the fixed or variable rate route must be made at the outset of the project. It is not possible at a later date to move from a variable rate reimbursement to a fixed rate reimbursement. Provided it is written into the loan offer, it is possible, however, to move after a period of years from a fixed rate reimbursement to a variable reimbursement rate. Should the loan be set up on a combination of fixed and variable rates, the basis of reimbursement will then be determined by the higher of the two loan ratios.

Variable rate loans – pros and cons

Since 1 April 1990 the variable rate cost rent reimbursement has been set on an annual basis. The formula currently being used by the Department of Health in setting the rate is to take the clearing bank's base rate at 1 April and add to this a margin of 1%. This takes no account of anticipated movements in interest rates over the next 12 months, which is when the reimbursement is payable. As a result, GPs will enjoy profit on the reimbursement rate when interest rates fall during the year and will be out of pocket in a year when interest rates are rising. As most surgery loans are taken out over a 20–25-year period, the variable rate route involves some risk of 'mismatch' during the term of the loan. Based on a loan of £500 000, the equivalent of a 1% movement in rates over a year would amount to a difference of £5000 to the practice as a profit or loss over the period. The main advantage under the variable rate option is that provided you give adequate notice to the lender, no early redemption penalty is payable. This avoids the potential problems that may arise when partnership changes occur where there are long-term fixed rates involved.

Fixed rate loan – pros and cons

The fixed rate reimbursement is reviewed quarterly by the Department of Health. The actual rate that will apply to a particular project is the fixed rate of reimbursement that is in force when tenders for the project are accepted. Once the rate has been agreed, it will continue at the same level until the practice moves to a notional rent.

Some lending sources will allow considerable flexibility as to when you lock into their fixed rate. This can be either at offer stage, acceptance of tenders, legal completion of the mortgage or, with the HA's permission, for a period after tenders have been accepted. This means that provided borrowers carefully plan the date of acceptance of tender, they should be able to lock into a fixed rate that matches or is an improvement on the reimbursement rate. Any saving that is made will help with the capital repayments or with funding any overspending in relation to the project. In recent years the Department of Health has tightened the margin when setting the fixed rate reimbursement, making it more difficult for GPs to match fixed-rate borrowing with the reimbursement rate. The date of acceptance of the tender can therefore be crucial to the overall project viability.

It is not always possible for GPs to be aware of all the intricacies involved when they accept their chosen building tender. It is therefore essential to seek the help of a cost rent specialist who understands the implications involved to appraise you of the fixed and variable rate facts and to assist you in making the right decision for your practice.

A fixed rate provides stability when interest rates are fluctuating and enables the practice to plan other financial commitments without the worry of an increase in existing outgoings.

Every three years or on completion of a major extension or refurbishment project, the cost or notional rent will be reviewed. At some future review date, when the notional rent exceeds the current cost rent, the reimbursement can be switched to a notional or current market rent which will produce a higher reimbursement amount.

With a fixed rate cost rent it is obvious when the time is right to switch to a notional rent. This is not so obvious with a variable rate reimbursement backed by a variable rate loan. In such circumstances should interest rates rise after the changeover, the practice could find itself out of pocket on its interest payment.

To protect against such movements in rates it is worth considering switching the loan to a fixed rate at the same time as the move to notional rent. If you match the fixed rate with the new notional rent, then your cash flow is secure for the next three years. The district valuer's (DV) view of the notional rent can be challenged if you are not in agreement with it. This is worth doing even in the early years, as should you be successful in raising the level of the reimbursement, it will be that increased figure that will be used as the threshold for the next review. This will eventually mean that you will reach the crossover point from cost to notional rent earlier than you would otherwise have done. It should be remembered, however, that on appeal the original amount of notional rent could be reduced.

The timing of the notional rent exceeding the cost rent will depend on the location of the property, availability of property in the area, and the localised inflation of rents and property values. In the past, notional rent has exceeded cost rent after nine years. Currently, with low inflation, a more realistic forecast would be 12 or 15 years. There has, however, been substantial variation either way in relation to the above timescales. In some cases it has been known for practices to be better off on a notional rent basis from day one. Falling interest rates may effect future trends.

Once a project has switched from cost rent to notional rent, it cannot then revert back to cost rent just because there is a change in interest rates. Current interpretation of the *Red Book* by DVs allows for movement in the notional rent both upwards and downwards at each triennial review. Once again it is of the utmost importance to seek expert advice before making a decision on whether or not the practice should switch to notional rent.

The single biggest drawback with fixed rate loans is the redemption penalty that may be incurred on early repayment. Some sources will charge a redemption penalty if the loan is repaid during the fixed rate term irrespective of the reinvestment rate. With such lenders there is normally an overall maximum of a number of months' interest or a flat percentage of the outstanding loan amount payable. This allows the practice to assess their maximum redemption liability at outset. Other sources will only charge a redemption penalty if the reinvestment rate is lower than the rate at which the original loan was taken out. Under such loans the penalty is the difference between the original fixed rate and the reinvestment rate multiplied by the capital outstanding, times the balance of the term.

The resulting figure is then discounted because the amount is being paid in advance as a lump sum. A separate formula is used for repayment and interest only loans. In theory the calculation is an actuarial one designed to leave the lender in a 'no lose' situation in the event of an early repayment of all or part of a loan. The reality is that it is possible for a lender, in an effort to protect their existing loan book and to dissuade borrowers from remortgaging to a cheaper source, to manipulate the reinvestment rate. To prevent this from happening to your practice, enlist the help of an expert when considering the repayment of all or part of the loan. Such penalties are indeterminable at the outset and can be very severe where there is a large differential between the original fixed rate and the reinvestment rate. Based on a fixed interest rate of 6.5% per annum and an outstanding loan balance of £500 000 with 15 or 20 years of the loan remaining, the penalty for each 1% differential at the redemption date would be £50 000 and £60 000 respectively. The penalty involved will be charged automatically, but some lenders, if requested, will give a discount on the amount outstanding if the reinvestment rate is higher than the original fixed rate.

Notional rent

Where reimbursement is paid on a notional rent basis the practice can fund the project by borrowing on either a fixed or a variable rate basis or any combination of the two. There are no overriding rules to push the borrower down a particular path; the rates chosen will be completely at the discretion of the practice.

Between the general election of 1997 and the beginning of 1998 a number of rate rises saw the variable rate at base-plus-one stand at 8%, the highest it had been for almost five years. On the other hand, long-term fixed rates stood at 6.5%, a 25-year low.

If rates can fluctuate so quickly in such a short timespan, what will happen over the next 20 years? With hindsight the argument for taking out a long-term fixed rate loan at around 6.5% is compelling. However, no matter how attractive long-term fixed rates may look, on a historical basis, the consensus of opinion is that when we join the European monetary union (EMU), interest rates will fall. The fact that at the end of 1998 the cost of long-term fixed rate money is low is based on the assumption that rates will be even lower in the future.

Considering the above, what is the answer for borrowers who want the security of a fixed rate? On the one hand, long-term fixed rates with the possibility of exorbitant redemption penalties can be a costly straightjacket, but the alternative worry of a return to variable rates of 16.75%, as in 1990, would play havoc with the practice's cash flow.

A viable alternative for those wishing to pursue the fixed rate cost rent or notional rent route would be a fixed rate of up to five years. This would provide the comfort and stability of a fixed rate in the short term and allow long-term fixed rates to settle after entry into EMU, before a decision needs to be made about locking in to the next fixed rate. If, in the interim, it was necessary to opt out of the short-term fixed rate in order to avail of a particularly attractive long-term fixed rate, the early repayment penalty would be considerably less than that applicable to someone switching from a long-term fixed rate of 6.5%.

For the more adventurous practices who wish to borrow in excess of £500 000 there are a number of interest rate hedging products available.

Interest rate swap

This is an agreement to exchange interest payments on a sum of money for a period normally up to 20 years. The frequency of the interest payments and the term can be tailored to the practice's needs, thus allowing accurate planning for the future. An interest rate swap takes the risk out of London Inter Bank Offer Rate (LIBOR) borrowing. Normally if you borrow at LIBOR plus a margin there is a risk that the underlying LIBOR rate will rise during the term of the loan. By entering into an interest rate swap the variable LIBOR rate can be exchanged for a fixed rate for up to 20 years of the loan. In lieu of LIBOR, the lending source is paid the pre-agreed fixed (swap) rate.

Swap rates are not always guaranteed to be cheaper than conventional fixed rates. It is, however, an option that should always be considered since there will be times when it can produce a significant rate advantage over fixed rates. One of the main advantages of an interest rate swap is that it is a stand-alone transaction which can be reviewed regularly and easily unwound at current market rates, should this prove advantageous to the practice.

Interest rate capping

This is another alternative to fixed rate lending which in certain circumstances may be used to give a greater degree of flexibility. As the name implies, a capped rate limits the maximum interest rate payable on any borrowing whilst allowing profit to be realised on any reduction in interest rates. Capped rates are normally for up to a maximum of five years, with the level of protection being tailored to meet the practice's specific requirements. The cost is a single up-front premium which can generally be added to the loan.

By introducing a 'collar', which is a combination of a cap and a floor which is the minimum rate payable on the loan, the amount of up-front premium payable can be structured to fit in with the cost or notional rent income stream. With interest rates set to fall as a result of entering into the EMU, a combination of swap, capped and collar rates may be a more attractive option than the standard fixed rates currently available.

Points to remember when undertaking a cost rent project

It is the DV's assessment of the value of the land that will be included in the cost rent calculation. Therefore, if you pay over and above that valuation, the practice will be funding the interest on the overspend from their own resources. Other pitfalls to look out for are hidden costs involved in acquiring a site, such as the planning permission being conditional on providing extra off-site car parking, the widening of the access road, and so on. Such costs are not normally allowed as an 'exceptional site cost'. Even when certain extras are allowed as 'exceptional site costs' they normally add very little value – if any – to the project, and the practice will still have to fund the extra capital repayment.

Where there is the probability of a vendor holding the practice to ransom on a purchase, it is worth employing a third party to acquire an option to purchase the site or the property involved. The option would normally be acquired for a limited period and be subject to planning permission, with any deposit being refundable in the event of the planning permission being refused. This approach can lead to substantial savings on the purchase price.

Should the practice have to purchase or extend an existing non-purpose-built property, consideration should be given to the ultimate resale value of the property at some future date, should it no longer be suitable for use as a surgery. For example, if a former residential property is purchased for, say, £300 000 and then extended and refurbished under a cost rent scheme at a further cost of £500 000, the underlying value as a residential property will increase very little. In fact, it would probably have decreased in value by the cost of the conversion back to a residential property. Assuming the property is almost fully cost-rented and continues to be run as a surgery, the project would, during that period, be financially viable for the practice. The problem arises if, say, 20 years down the line the practice outgrows the surgery and has to move to new premises. The new partners at that time will have bought in at whichever is the highest of the two options: either £800 000 (the total project cost) or the current market value.

If the property is then sold for £300 000 or its inflationary equivalent, a real loss of up to £500 000 will have been crystallised with all the current property owners losing out to varying degrees. This problem can be minimised by obtaining an improvement grant for as much of the work as possible. The partnership agreement should, under these circumstances, include a clause which would exclude the works paid for by the improvement grant from future valuations. The reverse could be true where a surgery has a much higher valuation for an alternative usage such as a commercial development site.

Where the land is being purchased from the local council, it is possible that they will only grant a long lease on the site and that it is conditional on the satisfactory completion of the building within a certain timescale. In such circumstances, the practice will normally have to proceed on the basis of a building agreement or agreement to lease. From a lending perspective, this does not offer the same security as a normal lease. In all such cases, before the building work commences your solicitor should liaise with both the council and the lender's solicitors with regard to the agreement and the lease which is to be eventually granted. Getting all the parties to agree acceptable terms can lead to frustrating time delays. The temptation to proceed without written confirmation from the council of the points agreed verbally should be avoided at all costs. In such circumstances, should the verbal agreements not materialise, the practice would be faced with having to accept a far more onerous lease than was first envisaged, or alternatively having to forfeit all its expenditure to date. It has been known in some cases for the borrower to have to undertake further expense to restore the site to its original state before returning it to the council.

While most freehold and long leasehold premises offer good prospects of a long-term return, this is not the case for short commercial leases with no assurance of the lease being extended at the end of its term. Such leases have very little value and, as a result, it is difficult to raise finance for such deals. If this is the only course of action available, the practice should approach the HA for a grant to purchase the lease with the balance being raised by way of unsecured loans from one of the high street banks.

In such circumstances the premises become a liability rather than an asset of the practice. Most lending sources will require the lease to have an unexpired term of at least 25 years at the end of the mortgage term before they would consider it a suitable collateral for a loan.

Possible pitfalls to consider prior to applying for a loan

- Change of bank manager could bring a change of attitude.
- Some lenders will insist on bank accounts either up front or in the future.
- The bank may wish to see the practice accounts on a regular basis and charge you for the privilege.

- The bank may not be in the market when future loans are required for buy-ins, extensions or refurbishment.
- Should you return to the bank for further funds during the building stage and there has been upward movement in fixed rates, you may be charged a higher rate on the extra amount required. To avoid this happening the point should be addressed at the outset of negotiations.
- If the bank at some future date thinks that they are overexposed due to a downturn in the property market, they may withdraw or restrict the practice's overdraft facilities for the day-to-day running of the surgery.
- Some lenders may lack expertise at local level to guide you through the cost rent maze or to liaise with the HA to sort out potential problems that may arise. In this scenario, the practice may experience complications during the initial stages of the project which can add to the overall cost. The appointment of an experienced team will minimise the possibility of this happening.
- The bank may have a minimum rate for variable rate lending.

Application procedures

Having assessed the marketplace and decided on a lending source you should submit a formal application as early as possible in order to have sufficient time to comply with any special requirements the lender may wish to enforce before money can be made available for the project.

The application should be supported, where possible, by a copy of the business plan that would have been submitted to the HA when enlisting their support; three years' practice accounts; details of the building works to be undertaken; and, where available, a letter from the HA confirming their support for the project, stating the amount of the cost/notional rent and any improvement grant that may be involved. Where an improvement grant is involved, it should include any specific conditions that are attached to it, and if none, that should also be stated.

The business plan should include appraisals under the following headings.

Current premises situation

- Facilities for patients

  - are the waiting areas adequate?

  - are there adequate toilet facilities, including disabled access?

  - can patient confidentiality be protected during discussions with the receptionist and the GP?

  - are there adequate rooms for ancillary practice staff to see patients?

- Staff facilities

  - are reception areas adequate?

  - is there a staff common room?

  - are there separate toilets for staff members?

  - is the patient record storage space easily accessible?

- Externally

  - are patient and staff parking facilities adequate?

  - is there proper access for the disabled? (This is a requirement by law)

  - are there adequate fire escapes? (This is also a requirement by law)

Planned premises improvements

Using similar headings to the above, state the proposed improvements and point out the benefit to the patients and the practice in each case.

Practice services

State the current services carried out and the proposed services that will be carried out from the new premises and the benefit this will give to the patients and staff in each case.

Distribution of the practice area and local community

This should include the list size and whether it will expand as a result of the new development.

Risk management

This should cover all the options available and the likely consequences of choosing that option. The following are considerations:

- expand on the existing site
- maintain the same building and do nothing
- restrict list size and/or reduce services
- assess alternative sites.

Give details of GPs involved in the project and whether or not it is intended to expand the number of partners in the future. The plan should also include a 'SWOT' analysis of the practice under the headings 'strengths, weaknesses, opportunities and threats'. The above list, whilst not exhaustive, gives examples of what should be covered in the plan.

Where the practice wishes to expand its list size and is therefore intending to build a surgery which will allow it to take on two or three new partners, an additional letter should be obtained from the HA confirming its long-term support for the project and endorsing the GPs' future plans for expansion of the partnership and confirmation that they will not reduce the cost rent if other GPs do not join the practice. Once the lending source has received its various requirements, it will normally issue a written loan offer within five working days. This loan offer will be subject to their standard conditions, and special conditions applicable to your particular project. It will also advise you if a survey is required and who is responsible for the survey fee.

Examples of some of the standard conditions

- Borrowers' names.

- Interest rates charged.

- Security required – because of the guaranteed income stream, the surgery premises will be sufficient security in most instances.

- Amount of loan agreed – in order to avoid having to apply for a further loan amount at a later date, you should include a continency amount of approximately 10% of the project cost.

- Interest roll-up facility. This is important as the cost or notional rent will not be paid by the HA until the building has been brought into use as a surgery.

- Repayment methods and term.

- Early repayment penalties.

- Default procedure.

- Property insurance – most lenders will charge a nominal fee if the insurance is not through their agency.

- Fees and costs.

- General terms and conditions.

- Minimum interest rate – this could be a major problem if rates fall sharply when we enter the EMU.

- Loans may be repayable on demand – this clause could cause problems in the future if the bank choose to call in the loan at a time when refinancing could be difficult.

- Regular reviews of securities which the practice will be charged for. At one of these reviews they could ask for additional security or call in the loan if they are not happy with the overall level of security at that time.

- There may be a clause which will allow the bank to dictate whether or not you can bring in new partners.

Examples of some of the special conditions

- Life insurance policies to be assigned.

- Improvement grants – this should include a statement to the effect that no early redemption penalties will be payable in respect of this type of early repayment.

- Second charges on residential properties – should a charge be required, you should negotiate it for a limited period if possible, or alternatively limit the extent of the second charge. In respect of the valuation of the residential property, most lending sources will accept a certificate of value as sufficient proof of value. The cost of the certificate should be nominal.

- Lease agreements – where third parties are to occupy part of the property, on completion the lending source will require that prior to legal completion you have in place at least a legally binding agreement to lease the portion of the building in question. The lease should be for a minimum of 20 years and should be approved by the lender's solicitors. On completion, the lender will normally take an assignment by way of a charge on the rents from the various tenants. This will allow them, in the event of default on the practice's part, to collect the rents directly from the tenants. In the first instance it will be your responsibility to collect the rent and pass on the required repayment to the lender.

When a loan is made to a number of partners, they shall be jointly and severally responsible for the loan. In some instances, an 'all monies charge' is involved, which can give the lender a floating charge over all the assets that come under their umbrella. This could include bank deposits and your residential property, should your residential mortgage be through the same source.

Another common problem which can cause a delay to completion is where there is a defective title to part of the property or land being offered as security. Most problems normally arise in relation to access and right of way. In such circumstances, the lender will normally require that a defective title indemnity policy be purchased.

The following information will be required by the underwriters in order that they may assess the risk:

- Where you already own the land, you will be required to sign a statutory declaration giving the history of the use of the right of way by you, as the owner. Any such declarations by previous owners that may be with the deeds which confirm usage over a longer period would considerably strengthen your case.

- Is the owner of the access way known?

- Is its use (with and without vehicles) without challenge, or objection, or payment of any kind?

- A copy of the site layout plans and confirmation from the architect, stating that he/she has inspected the planning file and that there were no objections to planning on the grounds of the access way, is necessary.

- Will the access be used in the future by both patients and members of the practice?

- Full development value of the site.

The indemnity premium will be paid by way of a one-off cost which can be included in the loan amount. In order to minimise the premium, you should supply the underwriter with as much up-front information as possible. The provision of such cover is very specialised and premiums can vary considerably. It is therefore worth asking a number of sources to quote for the business.

The loan offer will normally have a date by which it must be accepted. Failure to comply with this date may mean that the lender will vary the terms on offer. In order that the practice is in a position to accept the loan offer within the timescale, it is important that you allocate sufficient time to your solicitor for taking you through the various loan conditions stated in the offer. It cannot be overemphasised that you should be fully aware of all the conditions and their implications before committing yourself to the loan as it could prove very costly to untangle any disagreements that arise after legal completion. On acceptance of the loan offer, the solicitors acting for the borrower will proceed with the examination of title and any lease agreements that are involved. If title, together with valuation, prove satisfactory, the practice will be in a position legally to complete on the transaction. Any outstanding bills should be sent to your solicitor, and he or she will request payment of these direct to their firm with the initial tranche of money required to complete the loan.

Should a practice require funds before legal completion, this would be possible by way of a promissory note with funds again being made available through the solicitor on production of the necessary receipts and bills.

On completion, subsequent instalments will normally be advanced direct to the GP's bank account on production of original architect's certificates and bills as proof of the expenditure. Payment should be within five working days of the lender receiving the above. A separate bank account should be used for the surgery project.

This will help in the smooth running of the finances, and in the case of a cost rent scheme it will allow rolled up interest to be identified easily. Practical completion should coincide with the surgery being fully operational, since on that date the roll-up of interest within a cost rent scheme will cease and the cost rent will take over. If there is a time lag between practice completion and the surgery being brought into use, the practice will be responsible for the interest payable for that period.

On completion of the project any interest that has been rolled up within the project cost will be capitalised and added to the amount of the outstanding loan. With a cost rent scheme the amount of the rolled-up interest will be fully cost rented. The amount of the repayment to the lending source would be calculated and collected either direct from the HA or via the practice bank account.

Buying into surgery premises

Before purchasing a share in practice premises, a GP should look at the following:

- Current ownership and size of existing shares.

- Size of the share expected to be acquired, and when.

- Share of cost/notional rent.

- Value of the premises and what basis it was assessed on.

- Number and types of outstanding loans.

- Whether or not a new loan can be affected for the total share, and if not, will a share of the existing loans be taken over and, if so, on what terms. The terms and conditions attached to the existing loans and how they are currently being repaid could have an adverse effect on your cash flow.

- Will you be allowed to use the practice premises to secure the loan for your share of the purchase? If not, you may have difficulty raising the loan and may have to pay a higher rate of interest than you would normally have anticipated for a non-secured loan.

- Ensure that the partnership agreement adequately covers ownership of the premises and future dealings in them.

- The value of any surgery premises is the *current valuation minus the outstanding loans on the premises*. Do not fall into the trap of paying for a full share of current valuation without the partnership making the appropriate repayment of a proportion of the existing loans.

- Protect your interest by appointing your own solicitor and have your own survey carried out if you think the cost of your share is excessive.

- Is there a sale of 'goodwill'? If you think there is, challenge it via the MPC.

In the final analysis, you need to assess the net cost per annum of the purchase and ascertain whether it is a constant or an increasing one. If this figure is affordable you are then in a position to weigh up the effect on your future standing within the practice, based on whether or not you join in the ownership of the surgery premises.

5

The accountant's viewpoint

VALERIE MARTIN

When planning a new surgery development it is very easy to get carried away with the excitement of planning the appearance and practicalities of the building itself while possibly overlooking the fact that this development will form one of the greatest investments that GPs will undertake in their lifetimes. As such, it can provide a tremendous opportunity for profit but also a great risk of financial loss if the financial viability of the project is not carefully reviewed.

The review of the financial viability of the surgery as an investment entails:

- a critical review of the costs of the development compared to the ultimate value of the surgery on completion

- a review of the funding available in the form of grants and the utilisation of fundholding savings to reduce the cost to the GPs

- a review of the current VAT position in relation to the possible recovery of any VAT on construction costs

- a review of the eligibility of any of the expenditure for tax relief under the capital allowances system

- a review of the loan finance available and the optimum repayment method for the GPs

- considering the merits of fixed and variable rate interest loans and choosing the appropriate method for those GPs

- a calculation of the net annual cost to the GPs of owning the new surgery

- considering alternatives to the ownership of the surgery premises by the GPs.

This chapter will now look at each of these in detail.

A comparison of the development costs with the valuation on completion

It is important to remember that although the principal purpose of a new surgery development is to provide a modern surgery with all the facilities for the provision of full primary care to the patients, it is nevertheless a major investment for the doctors.

Before proceeding with the construction stage it is therefore essential to consider the anticipated value of the building on completion and compare this to the cost to the doctors.

The valuation of surgery premises has been the subject of considerable concern and debate over recent years and most GPs now accept that it is very rash to go ahead with building a surgery or extending and reconstructing an existing one where the cost exceeds the ultimate value. New partners are much more aware of the risks of a poor property investment and are unlikely to agree to buy in at a price which exceeds a reasonable valuation.

GPs who are able to use fundholding savings or improvement grants to reduce the net cost to themselves are fortunate as they only need to ensure that the valuation covers the net cost which is the limit of their exposure.

Valuation methods have moved on over the past couple of years from a very rigid interpretation of how surgeries should be valued to a more realistic approach.

It is nevertheless essential to start from the requirement of section 54 and schedule 10 of the National Health Service Act 1977. This makes it unlawful for NHS general medical practitioners to sell the goodwill of their medical practice, and the sale of a surgery premises for any consideration which in the opinion of the Medical Practices Committee (MPC) is substantially above the market value is deemed to be a sale of goodwill.

It is a criminal offence to contravene the terms of the Act and it is therefore absolutely essential that any value used in a transaction between GPs is based on a reasonable market value for those premises.

However, the rigid interpretation of the Act gave rise to valuers valuing surgery premises at their open market value on an alternative use basis and ignoring the use of the premises as a surgery. During the recession in the late 1980s and early 1990s when commercial property prices fell dramatically, valuing surgeries as if they were offices led to many GPs in theory having negative equity where the surgery loans exceeded the value of the premises. Retiring GPs were understandably unhappy to sell their share of the surgery at a loss when the reality of the investment to the doctors was often that the cost rent income stream exceeded the loan interest and the ownership of the premise therefore represented a real asset. If a new partner was able to buy in on the basis of the low alternative use valuation, their share of the cost rent income stream would have greatly exceeded their loan interest and provided them with a marvellous investment.

The obvious inequity of this position led to the Royal Institution of Chartered Surveyors (RICS) being asked to set up a working party to review the valuation of surgery premises. This has resulted in the issue of new guidelines to surveyors on the appropriate methods of valuing surgery premises.

It is now acceptable that valuers should value surgery premises as a surgery and not on an alternative use basis. This enables them to take account of the full floor area and the facilities offered in the surgery. This has also had the effect of increasing notional rent valuations.

It is also accepted that a method of valuation called 'depreciated replacement cost' (DRC) is an appropriate method for valuing surgeries on a change of partner. This method is based on considering what it would cost to build an identical surgery on an identical plot of land at the present time, and discounting the value for any improvements which would be required to comply with current health and safety requirements and also for any repairs and redecorations which are required.

Where a new surgery has been built efficiently and a fair open market value was paid for the land, the DRC on completion should match the actual cost. However, if the doctors have paid too much for the land or incurred additional construction costs due to inefficiencies or overpriced aesthetic features, then they could be faced with a valuation on completion which falls below the original cost. For this reason it is still not acceptable to value a surgery at the greater of original cost or market value in order to protect the original partners from suffering a loss, as such an excess value can still be deemed to constitute a sale of goodwill.

Valuers can, however, incorporate the value of the cost rent or notional rent income stream into the valuation of the surgery premises for transactions between partners. Nevertheless, they do not generally do this unless specifically instructed to do so in the partnership agreement. They are also advised in the RICS guidance notes not to use this method for valuations for loan security purposes despite the fact that most lenders place considerable importance on the level of cost or notional rent reimbursement in agreeing the amount of the loan.

In incorporating the cost or notional rent income stream into a valuation, the valuer would still need to consider the condition and suitability of the premises to modern GP practice, and not just base the value on, for example, the cost rent cost. This would not affect a new surgery but could affect the value of an older surgery which may have a high cost rent income stream but be in need of substantial alteration or repair. This would give rise to considerable forthcoming expenditure which would not result in any increase to the income stream. In such a situation the value could be less than the original cost rent cost.

The debate on the method of valuing surgery premises is still not closed as the MPC has still not given approval to any method of valuation which gives rise to a value in excess of the consideration which would have been expected if the premises had not previously been used as a medical practice. The RICS guidelines nevertheless give a common-sense approach which has been tacitly adopted and provides GPs with a reasonable value of their premises to compare with budgeted costs when building a new surgery or undertaking a redevelopment.

Availability of grants and the utilisation of fundholding savings

It is obviously advantageous to GPs to reduce the cost to themselves of any surgery development as much as possible. This can also help considerably to reduce or eliminate any potential problem arising from the value of the completed development being less than its cost to the GPs. This is particularly important in the case of extensions, which rarely increase the value of the premises by the full amount of the cost, even though they add considerable benefit to the working conditions of the GPs and the services that can be provided to the patients.

The following sources of funding are potentially available, although the first step is always to discuss the actual availability of cash with your particular health authority (HA) and the HA's approval always needs to be obtained prior to the expenditure being incurred.

Improvement grants

Improvement grants provide lump sum payments to the GPs toward the cost of extending or improving an existing surgery, and thus reduce the amount of the total cost which the doctors have to fund themselves. The full mechanics of improvement grants are set out in detail in Chapter 2 but in principle, between one-third and two-thirds of the cost can be covered by an improvement grant, or even up to 90% in Tomlinson areas where any Tomlinson money is still available.

At present, an extension funded partly by an improvement grant can still be fully valued for notional rent purposes and can therefore be particularly financially attractive to GPs. The availability of full notional rent on such surgeries has been debated from time to time and GPs should therefore review the current position with their HA before embarking on any redevelopment which relies on a full notional rent income stream to be financially viable. If the notional rent were restricted by the proportion of the total improvement grant to the total cost, this could significantly reduce the future income stream.

Fundholding savings

The other way to reduce the actual capital outlay on a new surgery or an extension or redevelopment is to use fundholding savings against the cost. This is only available for fundholders until 31 March 1999, after which time any unused fundholding savings will be passed on to the primary care group (PCG). The availability of such savings against any capital expenditure by the GPs when the funds are in the PCG is unclear at the time of writing, but it is evidently beneficial to use any savings within the practice in the final year of fundholding. It has been proposed that a ceiling of £90 000 be placed on the amount of fundholding savings that a practice can spend on premises and capital equipment in the year to 31 March 1999.

Where either an improvement grant or fundholding savings are used towards the cost of a surgery development and this results in the value on completion exceeding the cost net of grants and savings to the doctors, it is important that the doctors then decide whether future transactions should be based on the full value. This would effectively result in any future retiring partner withdrawing as profit his share of the grant or savings. Alternatively, if a valuation excluded the proportion of the premises funded by grants and savings, then the value of those remains in the practice for future partners. There is no guideline on this, or any ideal solution. However, whatever decision is reached it needs to be included in the partnership agreement. If the decision is to exclude the value of grants and savings then it may be advisable to include a clause whereby partners retiring under the terms of this agreement should be compensated by future partners if they subsequently change the basis of valuation in this respect.

VAT and surgery premises

Builders have to charge VAT on the costs of construction, alteration, redevelopment or extension of surgery premises. The professional costs of architects, quantity surveyors and similar professionals will also bear VAT. Many doctors would like to be able to reclaim these VAT amounts, but fear that it is impossible to do so, or that it would be unduly complicated to arrange.

It is true that Customs and Excise have made the recovery of VAT very difficult for those businesses whose income is wholly or mainly exempt from VAT (which includes the medical profession). However, there are some circumstances when the recovery of VAT on construction costs is permitted, and can easily be set in place.

Dispensing practices

The dispensing of drugs on NHS prescriptions is zero rated for VAT purposes. Many dispensing practices have taken the opportunity that this affords to register for VAT with Customs and Excise. They will then receive regular refunds of VAT from Customs and Excise on the purchase of the drugs for dispensing and most, if not all, of the VAT on the costs of running the practice. This would cover, for example, surgery upkeep and overheads; heat, light and power; computer costs; general consumables; telephone; and so on.

If building work is undertaken in the case of a dispensing practice which is registered for VAT, VAT on the construction costs will normally be partially recoverable. The expense will be treated as a 'common overhead' of the practice, and the recoverable proportion of the VAT will be based on the ratio of income received from the dispensing activity as a proportion of the total income of the practice. The exact calculation of this recoverable percentage will be as agreed with Customs and Excise based on the circumstances relating to the individual practice. The normal 'standard method' is to recover a proportion of the VAT on the 'common' costs that relate to both the dispensing and consulting activities of the practice. The 'standard method' calculates this proportion by taking the ratio of dispensing income as a percentage of the total income of the practice, and applying that percentage to the recovery of the VAT on the 'common' costs.

Thus, for dispensing practices, there is always the opportunity to recover part of the VAT on construction costs. Additional recoveries of VAT can be achieved by combining the 'dispensing' recovery with those methods described below.

Tenanted premises

Many practices may be able to offer parts of their premises for occupation by tenants receiving either a rental or service charge. It is possible to elect to charge VAT to those tenants on the rents or service charges in order to achieve VAT recovery on the construction costs.

Therefore, if tenants can be found who are prepared to pay VAT on their rents to the practice, the practice can recover VAT on the costs of the construction. The actual percentage recovery rate would have to be negotiated with Customs and Excise, but a simple method could be agreed, for example one based on the floor area occupied by the tenants. In this way, the VAT recovery of the costs of construction would be the same percentage as the area of the building to be occupied by the tenants who were going to pay VAT on their rents to the practice.

Methods could also be agreed which took account of any shared part of the premises (e.g. waiting rooms, reception areas, toilets, etc.), which were to be shared by both the practice and the tenants, and a portion of the VAT relating to those areas could also be recovered.

It is not possible to charge VAT on rents to a 'connected' tenant under the circumstances described below. A 'connected' tenant is defined in the Taxes Act as someone who is one of the partners in the practice, or a relation of one of the partners, or a director of an associated company.

This will then mean that those rents to a 'connected' tenant will remain exempt from VAT, causing a restriction in the recovery of VAT on the construction costs, the restriction being based on the 'partial exemption' percentage calculation. This is the percentage that is either based on the ratio of 'taxable' income to the total income of the practice, or on the floor areas occupied by tenants paying VAT on their rents, or any other method agreed with Customs and Excise. In the 'standard' (income-based) method, the 'taxable' income would include the rents to 'unconnected' tenants, on which VAT was being charged, plus any dispensing income received (if the practice was a dispensing practice). For a non-dispensing practice, which did not have high levels of 'taxable' income, it would be much more beneficial to agree an apportionment of the VAT on the construction costs based on a floor area basis rather than an income basis. However, individual circumstances do differ, and each case should be considered on its own merits before the method of apportionment is agreed with Customs and Excise.

The restrictions on electing to charge VAT on rents

Rentals to connected tenants must remain exempt from VAT in the following circumstances:

- where the costs of construction (or refurbishment) exceed £250 000

- where the tenant is a 'connected person' (as defined in the Taxes Act)

- where the (connected) tenant is engaged in a business activity that is wholly or mainly exempt from VAT.

When these rents have to be VAT exempt, the VAT on the development costs will have to be apportioned, and a fair and reasonable method should be agreed with Customs and Excise. The method to be agreed can be based on the income ratios of the practice, or the floor areas to be occupied by tenants who are paying VAT on their rents, or any similar method.

The different methods available can result in substantially different levels of VAT recovery, so the most advantageous method should be calculated prior to commencement of the project. It is not usually possible to change your method of VAT recovery retrospectively.

Development companies

Practices can develop new surgeries as a partnership, or they may choose to establish a development company. A development company would not be able to charge VAT on the rents to a connected practice if the conditions above apply. The development company can charge VAT to unconnected tenants, and will need to apportion its VAT recovery on the costs of the construction project accordingly.

The normal 'standard' method of apportionment is to apportion the VAT on the construction costs in the same ratio as relates to the income of the development company, that is to say, taking taxable income as a percentage of total income. Sometimes the ratio can result in a higher taxable level of income in the year of construction as for VAT purposes, the level of recovery depends on the income received in each year ending on 31 March.

The ratio of recovery in the first year can be disproportionate depending on how near to 31 March the new surgery is occupied, and how much of the income for the period from the completion of construction up to the first 31 March is taxable as opposed to exempt. For example, if an unconnected tenant pays rent plus VAT prior to 31 March, and that is the only source of rental income received by the development company in that tax year, the company will be regarded as 'fully taxable' for VAT purposes in that year.

The development company, being 'fully taxable' in the VAT year, could then recover all the VAT in that year on the costs of construction. Customs and Excise would regard any such full recovery as disproportionate, because the surgery will actually thereafter be used to generate both taxable and exempt rents. This disproportionate rate of initial recovery is compensated for by the operation of the capital goods adjustment scheme, which is described below.

It is therefore possible for the development company to recover *all* the VAT on the costs of construction if no exempt income is received by it in the year of construction (i.e. the 12 months prior to 31 March). This is despite the fact that exempt rents are due to be received from the 'connected' tenant, being the practice, in the following VAT year (i.e. after 31 March).

This level of recovery in the initial year of construction will need to be reviewed over the following 10 years according to the rules of the capital goods adjustment scheme, as described below.

Capital goods adjustment scheme

If VAT is reclaimed on a construction or refurbishment project that has cost over £250 000, then adjustments to the recoverable percentage must be made for the next 10 years if the recoverable percentage fluctuates.

The recoverable percentage to be used for each of the adjustment years is the 'annual' partial exemption recovery rate applicable to the non-attributable ('common') input tax of the developer. This calculation is complicated and normally requires specialist advice prior to its implementation. However, once the annual partial exemption formula is set up, the percentage calculation follows a standard pattern and merely requires the insertion of the figures for the relevant year.

This is obviously extremely complicated and it is therefore essential to seek individual expert advice before embarking on such a scheme. Indeed, in all matters of partial exemption and VAT recovery for surgery construction projects, seeking professional advice at an early stage can be very beneficial. A good VAT consultant could assist you in structuring the project in such a way that significant VAT recoveries are achieved.

The rules set out above are those applicable at the time of writing, but VAT legislation does change from time to time, so before embarking on any project it is essential to receive current expert advice.

Eligibility for tax relief under the capital allowances system

Tax relief is not available on the cost of the construction of the building itself. However, capital allowances are available on certain expenditure on fixtures and fittings within the surgery which are sometimes provided by the builder as built-in fitments. It is therefore essential to provide your accountant with a copy of the complete builder's specification detailing each and every item of expenditure so that any qualifying items can be recognised and the tax relief claimed.

The general rule is that items only qualify for capital allowances if they pass the purpose or function test. However, an asset is not considered to serve a qualifying function if its principal purpose is to insulate or enclose the interior of the building, or to provide an interior wall, floor or ceiling of a permanent nature.

Expenditure which is likely to qualify will include:

- Space- or water-heating systems, powered systems of ventilation, air cooling or air purification.

- Manufacturing or processing equipment, storage equipment, display equipment, counters, checkouts and similar equipment. This category will cover the reception desk and integral built-in equipment.

- Lifts, hoists, escalators and any moving walkways. However, the shafts or other structures in which the lifts, hoists, etc. are installed are excluded as being part of the structure of the building itself.

- Sound insulation if provided to meet the specific requirements of the business.

- Computer, telecommunications and surveillance systems, including their wiring and any other links.

- Burglar alarm systems.

- Sprinkler equipment and any other equipment for extinguishing or containing fire, and fire alarm systems.

- Wash basins, sinks, baths, showers, sanitary ware and similar equipment.

- Cookers, washing machines, dishwashers, refrigerators, freezers, etc.

- Furniture and furnishings.

- Advertising signs, displays, etc.

- Partition walls, where moveable and intended to be moved in the course of the business. It is not enough for them just to be moveable.

Timing of tax relief under the capital allowances system

Tax relief is available on qualifying expenditure in the 'basis period'. This is basically the accounting period, so if accounts are prepared for the year ended 30 June 1999 then any qualifying expenditure in that period will be brought into the capital allowances computation for that period and tax relief given initially in 1999/2000 and subsequent years. The capital allowances are treated as an expense of the accounting period to arrive at the taxable profits to be allocated between the partners.

Adjusted profit for year ended 30 June 1999	£280 000
Deduct capital allowances	£40 000
Profits chargeable to tax in 1999/2000	£240 000

Capital allowances are generally available at 25% per annum on the qualifying expenditure and this relief is known as the writing down allowance. However, in the 1997 Budget, the Chancellor announced a special first-year allowance set at 50% for expenditure incurred in the period from 2 July 1997 to 1 July 1998. In the 1998 Budget the Chancellor announced that the first-year would be continued for a further year set at 40% for expenditure incurred between 2 July 1998 and 1 July 1999. After the first year, allowances will be given on a reducing balance basis at 25% per annum.

For example, if a GP practice incurred qualifying expenditure on its new surgery development of £80 000 in its year ended 30 June 1999, relief would be given as shown in the table below. It does therefore take quite a few years to obtain tax relief on the full cost of the expenditure as can be seen from this example where, after a further 12 years, the balance of the expenditure still not relieved would be down to £691, so effectively obtaining near-full tax relief after 15 years.

	Surgery pool	Allowance
Year ended 30 June 1999		
Additions	£80 000	
First-year allowance (FYA) (40%)	(£32 000)	£32 000
Written down value (WDV) at 30 June 1999	£48 000	
Year ended 30 June 2000		
Written down allowance (WDA) at 25%	(£12 000)	£12 000
WDV at 30 June 2000	£36 000	
Year ended 30 June 2001		
WDA at 25%	(£9000)	£9000
WDV at 30 June 2001	£27 000	
Year ended 30 June 2002		
WDA at 25%	(£6750)	£6750
WDV at 30 June 2002	£20 250	

Loan finance and the optimum repayment method

The various types of loans and repayment methods are covered in detail in Chapter 4. The important deciding factor in choosing the type of loan and method of repayment best suited to you is to review your investment in the surgery premises as part of your overall investment strategy.

The principal point to remember is that tax relief at your top rate of tax is only available on loans to the partnership or sole practitioner or to individual partners where the loan is for the introduction of partnership capital. Therefore in reviewing your individual borrowing requirements it is important to ensure that wherever possible you take out loans for business purposes rather than loans for personal borrowings, including home mortgages. This also means that it is preferable to use funds to repay personal borrowings rather than accelerating the repayment of business loans.

Many GPs try to repay their surgery loans by the anticipated time of their retirement. However, this is not necessary unless the proceeds from the sale of the share in the surgery will be required to fund the individual's retirement in the absence of sufficient pension provision. Even in that position the GP may be better advised to review the possible ways of topping up the NHS superannuation pension and consider the timing of the repayment of the loan as part of this overall investment strategy.

Partnership loans versus personal loans for partnership capital

Sole practitioners can only obtain loans in their own name and claim the interest as a business expense in their accounts and are therefore unaffected by this consideration. However, GPs who are in partnership have the choice of either all joining together and obtaining a single loan to the partnership or of each obtaining individual loans for partnership capital.

Under the preceding-year-basis tax system there was a considerable advantage to the partners in taking out personal loans for partnership capital rather than a partnership loan to fund large borrowings for surgery premises. This was mainly tax driven and enabled them to obtain tax relief on the interest actually paid in the year rather than being given tax relief almost two years later when the accounts profit was taxed. It was particularly beneficial in the transition to the new tax system in 1996/97 when, effectively, tax relief on 12 months' loan interest was lost with partnership loans but full tax relief was available on all the interest paid on personal loans for partnership capital.

Under the new current-year basis of taxation there is a much shorter timescale between incurring partnership expenditure and obtaining tax relief on it. With a 30 June year end, tax relief would be obtained in 1999/2000 on expenditure incurred in the year ended 30 June 1999. With a 31 March year end, tax relief is effectively available on an actual year basis as tax relief is due in 1998/99 on expenditure incurred in the year ended 31 March 1999. This is identical to the tax relief on personal loans for partnership capital where tax relief is given in 1998/99 for eligible loan interest incurred in the year ended 5 April 1999.

The acceleration of the tax relief is therefore no longer a major consideration but personal loans may still be favoured where the GPs want the maximum flexibility in their borrowings with partners having different repayment methods and different loan periods to suit their individual needs. However, even this degree of flexibility can often be provided within a partnership loan by some lenders at present.

The only other consideration relates to pension planning. Loan interest in partnership loans reduces a GP's share of taxable profits which form the basis of the net relevant earnings for personal pension contribution purposes. However, with personal loans for partnership capital, the tax relief on the interest is claimed via the personal tax return and therefore the interest does not reduce the calculation of net relevant earnings. This enables a greater amount to be paid into a personal pension contribution and qualify for tax relief at that individual's top rate of tax. This is only of benefit to GPs who make personal pension contributions in addition to their superannuation contributions and in this case, this may be a relevant deciding factor.

However, for most GPs the advantages of the simplicity of a partnership loan and lack of complications on partner changes may weigh the balance in favour of a partnership loan. With personal loans for partnership capital it is necessary for a retiring partner selling his or her share of the surgery premises to repay his or her personal loan and then the new incoming partner has to take out a new loan. This obviously incurs some bank charges and land registry fees registering the new loan. However, most importantly, a retiring partner will no longer qualify for tax relief on the interest on the personal loan for partnership capital from the date of retirement as he or she is no longer a partner in the practice. It is therefore crucial that a retiring partner with a personal loan sells the share of the surgery premises on retirement, whereas a partner whose funding is in the form of a partnership loan does not need to be bought out so quickly. The loan interest on the whole partnership loan will still continue to be a qualifying expense in the practice accounts and the retired partner can just be paid the excess of the cost or notional rent over the loan interest, or pay any shortfall to the practice, until the sale of the premises goes through. Alternatively, continuing partners can assume responsibility for paying the share of the loan interest and in return keep the income stream, and the actual sale transaction can go through when the new partner is due to buy in, which may be a year or so later. This flexibility could not be achieved in the case of a personal loan without loss of tax relief or incurring costs.

Fixed versus variable rate interest loans

Loan finance for GPs funding new surgery developments is readily available at present, with several lending institutions offering very competitive rates for GPs. The reason GPs can borrow at such favourable rates compared to many other professionals is because the cost and notional rent schemes effectively fund the financing of the loan interest in the short term and ultimately the repayment of the loan, and therefore make GPs blue-chip customers in the eyes of the lenders.

So GPs can fairly easily negotiate favourable interest rates and their main decision will be whether to choose a fixed or a variable rate loan. The merits and downsides of the two types are covered in detail in Chapter 4 but the principal deciding factors are as follows:

- If the loan is obtained on a variable rate basis then the cost rent will be a variable rate cost rent. This is only adjusted annually, taking the clearing bank's base rate at 1 April and adding 1%. There is therefore a degree of exposure in that if interest rates rise in the year, the loan interest will increase but the cost rent reimbursement will remain at the same level. Alternatively, however, a profit can be achieved if interest rates fall in the year.
- If the loan is obtained on a fixed rate basis then the cost rent will also be on a fixed rate. The fixed rate that will apply to the cost rent is the fixed rate in force when the tenders for the project are accepted. There is some flexibility in the timing of when to lock into the fixed rate on the loan interest, being either at the offer stage, acceptance of tenders or legal completion of the mortgage, and it can therefore be possible, with good advice, to lock into a higher rate of cost rent reimbursement than the fixed rate applicable to the loan and thus make a profit on this.
- A fixed rate provides stability and certainty when interest rates are fluctuating. If the cost rent covers the whole cost of the surgery then a fixed rate gives total certainty and eliminates worry about interest rates. Even if the rate later appears high compared to current rates, the interest is fully covered by the equally high rate of cost rent reimbursement. However, if the actual cost of the project is greater than the cost rent cost then the GPs will have to fund the interest on the balance of the loan in excess of the cost rent. If this is on a fixed rate basis which later turns out to be higher than available variable rates, then this is a real cost to the doctors and could be a deterrent to a new partner joining in the loan. Conversely, a low fixed interest rate would be very attractive, so there is no easy solution and individual advice is needed at the time the loan is taken out.
- When a fixed interest rate loan is redeemed early there is a penalty for early redemption. This can be very high if interest rates are significantly lower at the time of redemption and this accordingly restricts flexibility. In the case of a variable rate

loan there should be no early redemption penalty so long as adequate notice is given to the lender. This is generally no more than three months' notice and in some cases just one month.

- Where GPs are in receipt of notional rent reimbursement, care needs to be taken with a variable rate loan as fluctuations in interest rates affect the cost of the loan interest but are not reflected in the reimbursement. Sudden interest rate rises can therefore cause considerable concern.

Review of the net annual cost of owning the surgery premises

In deciding whether or not a surgery is affordable, GPs need to avoid the trap of being put off by the sheer size of the numbers involved. An investment per individual GP of as much as £200 000 or even more may seem daunting but the actual affordability will depend upon the net annual outlay. It is only the actual net annual outlay which will have an effect on the GP's net disposable income and hence lifestyle.

This net annual cost to the GPs is calculated by comparing the share of the cost or notional rent received by the doctor with his or her loan interest and either capital repayments or endowment premiums in the case of an endowment mortgage. For example, if Doctor Wiseman's share of the cost of a new surgery development amounts to £140 000 and this is to be fully funded by a repayment loan, then his position may be as illustrated overleaf.

In this case, from a cashflow point of view, Dr Wiseman would need to fund the net cost of £1092 pa or £91 per month.

However, the capital repayment element of the outgoings really relates to the purchase of the investment and represents transferring one asset, being cash, into another asset, being ownership of the surgery premises. This still needs to be funded from a cashflow point of view but so long as the surgery is being purchased at a realistic value and represents a reasonably sound investment, then this capital repayment element of the cost does not diminish the GP's overall wealth.

Share of cost rent		£10 500
Less: interest	£10 160	
capital repayments	£1432	
		£11 592
Net annual outlay		(£1092)

In the above example the cost rent more than covers the loan interest and is in fact making a contribution towards the capital repayment of £340 pa.

Therefore although £140 000 may seem a large sum to borrow, particularly for a young GP who may also be in the process of buying a new house in the area, the investment in the ownership of the surgery premises would in this case represent a reasonable investment at very little cost to the doctor.

Alternatives to the ownership of the surgery premises by the GPs

In some cases the doctors in a practice may not be keen on becoming involved in surgery ownership. This may be for various reasons: a misconception regarding the actual cost to the GPs, or they do not have a long-term commitment to stay in the practice and therefore do not wish to be involved in a joint investment with their partners, or because they are concerned that properties in their particular area may not be an attractive investment.

It is important to review the actual reason why the GPs themselves do not wish to own the surgery premises in order to find the appropriate solution. If it is purely a misconception regarding the costs of surgery ownership then it is a matter of first discussing the overall financial position with a specialist GP accountant and in particular ascertaining the net annual cost to the doctors of owning the surgery. This may then show that, in fact, the surgery is an attractive investment, and the doctors may then wish to proceed.

However, if the calculations indicate that the proposed surgery is not financially viable then it may be necessary to go back to the drawing board and discuss matters again with the architect to try to redesign a surgery which will be financially attainable. It is important to acknowledge that if a surgery is not financially viable for the GPs themselves to develop then it probably will not be an attractive investment for anyone else to develop and therefore the possibility of renting the surgery from a property investment company may not be a realistic alternative.

The situation which is best suited to renting or private finance initiative funding is where the doctors do not wish to be property owners due to the temperament of the partners and possible frequent partner changes.

Private finance initiative

The private finance initiative (PFI) was launched by the last government and has made a few tentative steps into funding GP premises. However, to date it has very much been renting under another name. A true PFI project would have the developer not only owning the surgery premises but also managing the unit, controlling the overheads and even providing the staff. They would therefore be bringing a management expertise as well as taking the risks of the property ownership.

In the very few PFI projects which have so far been undertaken with regard to surgery developments, these have been in respect of large surgeries or primary healthcare resource centres. In these projects the GPs may have considered that the projects were too great an investment and risk for them to undertake personally or that sufficient funding was not available under the traditional cost rent and notional rent methods of surgery funding. In these cases PFI may be an appropriate alternative whereby an independent developer would undertake the development, working with the GPs on the design, and then lease the completed centre to the GPs.

The leases are generally for periods of 25 years with regular three-yearly rent reviews. The rent on the main part of the surgery used for general medical services purposes is reimbursable by the HA so long as it is at a current open market rent. For this reason upward-only rent reviews should be viewed with caution as they can lead to the rent being increased above the open market rent which the HA will reimburse. The remainder of the surgery or primary care resource centre would need to generate sufficient income to cover its costs, including the rent.

This is therefore very much just renting under another, more fashionable name. It should be noted that a PFI developer will only be interested in the surgery if they consider that the site has good development potential and the developers will be looking to recover their investment over the 25-year period. So PFI does not provide the panacea for a surgery development which does not appear to be financially attractive to the GPs themselves.

The present government is keen on promoting PFI in primary care and is currently reviewing the possibility of putting together consortia of GPs and private developers. The intention is to consider taking groups of up to 30 surgery developments in a geographical area and offering them as a package to private contractors. If GPs are interested in the PFI route they may therefore wish to discuss this possibility with their HA, but the idea has not yet been widely taken up by private developers as the prospect of developing a large number of fragmented sites is not necessarily financially attractive to them. However, this could become the way forward, when combined with the new PCGs, for GPs for whom property investment is not an attractive prospect however potentially profitable it may be.

Appendix A
SFA definition for minimum standards

Minimum standards

'51.10 Premises will not be accepted under the Scheme unless the accommodation provided is deemed adequate by the HA following a visit taking into account the circumstances of the practice and having regard to the need for:

i   ease of access to premises and movement within them, bearing in mind the needs of elderly and disabled people, including those who are wheelchair bound, and parents with young children

ii   a properly equipped treatment room, where provided, and a properly equipped consulting room for use by the practitioner and also, where appropriate, by nurses and other members of the primary healthcare team, with adequate arrangements to ensure the privacy of consultations and the right of patients to personal privacy when dressing or undressing, either in a separate examination room or in a screened off area around an examination couch within the treatment room or the consulting room

iii the practitioner, staff and patients to have convenient access including wheelchair access, to adequate lavatory and washing facilities. Practitioners should have a wash basin in their consulting room and if not, then immediately adjacent

iv adequate internal waiting areas with enough seating to meet all normal requirements and provision, either in the reception area or elsewhere, for patients to communicate confidentially with reception staff including over the telephone

v the premises, fittings and furniture to be kept clean and in good repair, with adequate standards of lighting, heating and ventilation

vi adequate fire precautions, including provision for safe exit from the premises, designed in accordance with the Building Regulations agreed with the local fire authority

vii adequate security for records, prescription pads, pads of doctors' statements and drugs

viii where the premises are used for minor surgery, a suitable room and equipment for the procedures for which the room and equipment is used.'

Appendix B
Chronological sequence of steps to be taken

Part I

These are the preliminary steps to be taken before substantial costs are committed to check the overall viability of the project. All the team members should be specialists in their particular fields.

Approval in principle:

- general support for the practice move   Health Authority
- guidelines about the area within
  which to move
- funding availability

Preliminary advice before embarking on the   Solicitors
scheme: Accountants
                                                 IFA
- to ensure the Partnership and the
  Partnership Agreement is sound
- to ensure the financial standing of the
  Partnership is sound
- to consider the future impact on the
  Partnership in both legal and financial
  terms

Produce a Feasibility Study for the purposes of enabling the Health Authority to determine whether it can facilitate the GPs' proposed scheme	Health Authority Solicitors Accountants Architect
Consider whether to: • develop building already owned by the Partners • find and develop either an existing building or greenfield site	Surveyor Architect Solicitors Accountant
Identify a specific site and negotiate the proposed Heads of Terms	Surveyor Solicitors
Prepare Concept Proposal to include: • planning issues • outline design • site conditions • preliminary costing issues	Architect
Work up Business Plan • Consideration by Health Authority of improved facilities and/or services to be available leading to written offer of support and funding, e.g. grant, cost/ notional/rent reimbursement	Health Authority
Check effect of nature of the proposed scheme on the Partnership to include in particular the impact of valuation issues for the future	Solicitors Accountants

Check the availability of a funding source for the proposed scheme	IFA
If possible, enter into an option to acquire the site. NB: this may not be available but if it can be achieved, it reduces the exposure of the risk that the seller of the site will refuse to proceed after heavy costs have been incurred under Part II below	Solicitors
Application for outline planning consent	Architect

Part II

At this stage the scheme is viable in principle and you can proceed to work up the detail. However, it will be apparent that a number of different specialists will be involved simultaneously with the resultant commitment to costs.

Health authority	Specialist architect	Specialist solicitors	Specialist accountants	Specialist IFA
		Advice on offer of funding		Written offer of funding
• Liaise to keep abreast of developments and to ensure ongoing support	• Application for detailed planning permission • Detailed design and specification • Agreement of form of building contract • Agreement of terms of appointment with design consultants and collateral warranties • Going out to tender	• Investigation of title • Negotiation of agreement for lease and lease (if appropriate) • Approval and negotiation of building contract • Approval and negotiation of collateral warranties • Variation to partnership agreement	• Advice generally throughout this period	• Advice on repayment vehicles and their tax implications

Health authority	Specialist architect	Specialist solicitors	Specialist accountants	Specialist IFA
	• Appointment of the design team to include the planning supervisor • Confirmation that detailed planning permission is available together with building regulation approval [and fire approval]	• Preparation of engrossment of contract for signature • Letter to health authority containing statement that GPs are ready to exchange and will be relying upon the health authority offer of support and funding in doing so together with terms of any conditions attached and a declaration that the health authority will be deemed to have approved the conditions unless a response is received within a specified number of working days	• Final approval of all financial implications	• Acceptance of offer of funding: make sure that all the loan conditions have been fulfilled

Part III

Final reports in preparation for exchange of contracts.

Health authority	Specialist architect	Specialist solicitors	Specialist accountants	Specialist IFA
	• Return of acceptable tender • Approval of contractor by the health authority • Accept the tender • Enter into the building contract	• After any deadline imposed in the letter to the health authority has passed: exchange of contracts for purchase/lease of the site		• Advice on the timing of accepting the tender and its implications, especially with regard to fixed rates

Part IV

Preparation for completion.

		• If freehold/long leasehold acquisition: pre-completion searches, draw down of funding		• Liaison re drawdown of funding • Building and contents insurance

Part V

Completion of freehold.

Health authority	Specialist architect	Specialist solicitors	Specialist accountants	Specialist IFA
	• Building contract let and works commence • Completion of works and issue of Certificate of Practical Completion	• Legal completion of purchase • Legal completion of funding documentation		

Part VI

Completion of leasehold.

- Final DV approval of the completed project and final assessment of the level of cost/notional/rent reimbursement

- Post completion snagging
- Correction of defects

- Legal completion of grant of lease

1 It is essential to report any changes in the circumstances to the scheme to all relevant parties listed above.

2 The suggested chronology is of general application only and it is essential that expert specialist advice be sought in order to determine the best way forward in any given scheme.

Index

Milton Keynes UK
Ingram Content Group UK Ltd.
UKHW031150141024
449569UK00024B/910